WITHDRAWN

2 3 JUN 2021

Traffickers

Drug trafficking is the fastest growing area of international crime. In Britain, it has stimulated the modernisation of policing and propelled us half-way towards a national police force. What is the reality of the crime which stimulates such a far-reaching response?

Traffickers rejects the conventional idea that drug trafficking is dominated by large criminal organisations. Big traffickers, the mafia, cartels – these are myths, nourishing the popular imagination and stimulating advances in law enforcement. Using the words of those involved, both the dealers and the detectives, *Traffickers* exposes the diversity of drug trafficking today, and provides an account of how police operations work. It includes:

* accounts of the development of drug markets from the 1960s to the 1990s
* a discussion of the evolution of new policing methods, including secret 'intelligence development' operations
* insider views on the development of a national detective agency for Britain
* a challenging look at the processing and sentencing of drug traffickers
* extended extracts from a hitherto unpublished and confidential report from the Association of Chief Police Officers.

Essential reading for students and professionals in the field of criminology, *Traffickers* will also be of interest to all those concerned about major developments in policing which will affect us all.

College of Ripon & York St. John

3 8025 00269099 1

111609

Traffickers

Drug markets and law enforcement

Nicholas Dorn, Karim Murji
and Nigel South

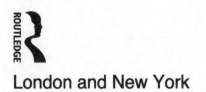

COLLEGE OF RIPON
AND YORK ST. JOHN
YORK CAMPUS
LIBRARY

ROUTLEDGE

London and New York

First published in 1992
by Routledge
11 New Fetter Lane, London EC4P 4EE

Simultaneously published in the USA and Canada
by Routledge
a division of Routledge, Chapman and Hall Inc.
29 West 35th Street, New York, NY 10001

© 1992 Nicholas Dorn, Karim Murji and Nigel South

Typeset by Selectmove Ltd, London
Printed and bound in Great Britain by
Mackays of Chatham PLC, Chatham, Kent

All rights reserved. No part of this book may be reprinted or
reproduced or utilized in any form or by any electronic,
mechanical, or other means, now known or hereafter
invented, including photocopying and recording, or in any
information storage or retrieval system, without permission in
writing from the publishers.

British Library Cataloguing in Publication Data
Dorn, Nicholas
   Traffickers: drug markets and law enforcement.
   1. Great Britain. Criminal investigation. Drug investigation
   I. Title II. Murji, Karim III. South, Nigel 363.450941

Library of Congress Cataloging in Publication Data
   Dorn, Nicholas.
   Traffickers: drug markets and law enforcement / Nicholas Dorn,
   Karim Murji, and Nigel South.
   p. cm.
   Includes bibliographical references and indexes.
   1. Drug traffic – Great Britain. 2. Narcotics, Control of – Great
   Britain. 3. Narcotic laws – Great Britain. I. Murji, Karim, 1960–II.
   South, Nigel. III. Title.
   HV5840.G7D57 1991
   363.4'5'0941–dc20

                                               91–8741
                                                CIP

ISBN 0–415–03536–8
     0–415–03537–6 (pbk)

Contents

Acknowledgements

We cannot for reasons of confidentiality name many of the people who have helped us by facilitating access to situations, people or information.

We wish to thank the traffickers, ex-traffickers, police informers and others who gave us their perspectives. We interviewed eighty people falling into this broad category, most of whom had personal experience of trafficking, twenty-five of whom were seen in prisons. Throughout the book, no trafficker or ex-trafficker is named and disguises have been provided in many cases.

For consistency's sake, as far as the enforcement agencies are concerned, we name organisations but not individuals. The Home Office and several prison governors and their staff helped us to gain access to convicted persons who wished to talk. We wish to acknowledge the help given us by the Association of Chief Police Officers, who also kindly granted us permission to include as an Appendix extracts from their hitherto unpublished 'Broome Report' on drug enforcement. The National Drugs Intelligence Unit (NDIU) and some of its staff introduced us to the rudiments of drugs intelligence in practice. Together with the Crack Intelligence Unit, staff of the NDIU and local officers helped us to piece together an understanding of intelligence development (though we alone are responsible for the interpretations we have placed on the incomplete information available to us). Officers in Regional Crime Squads and their drugs wings, in the Metropolitan Police Central Drugs Squad and in city and county forces and asset confiscation teams took time to describe their operations to us. We are grateful to Notting Hill police (an identity that the material makes impossible to disguise) for sharing with us their account of recent developments in policing street markets. Luckily, we were able to learn something about importations from police officers, imprisoned persons and other sources, so the relatively lukewarm response of HM Customs and Excise did not greatly inconvenience us.

This work would not have been possible without the support of the Sainsbury family charitable trusts who, rather against the odds, funded the work. The Institute for the Study of Drug Dependence provided the environment for research. Its Director, Jasper Woodcock, the staff of the Institute's reference library and other colleagues were unstinting in their assistance throughout the study. Andrew Fraser, Mark Gilman and Kamlesh Patel went out of their way to help us on several occasions. Michael Keith shared information from his research in Notting Hill. Geoff Pearson has been a good friend and sympathetic critic, David Downes, Gerry Mars and Robert Reiner gave us support when it was needed, and Mike Woodiwiss and Philip Bean did their best to divert us from completion of this book.

Introduction

Drug trafficking[1] is probably the fastest growing area of international crime – setting aside corporate crimes such as environmental pollution, degrading the food chain, fraud and so on. And, of all areas of crime control, drug trafficking has been at the forefront of stimulating developments in terms of legislation and the organisation of law enforcement. Domestically, confiscation of the proceeds of trafficking provides the clearest example, with the passage of the Drug Trafficking Offences Act 1986. That innovation has since found its way into other branches of law, asset confiscation provisions being extended to all other crimes with a gain of more than £10,000 by the Criminal Justice Act 1988. Similar powers are also provided for in the Prevention of Terrorism Act 1989.

Internationally, drug trafficking has been one of the two main spurs to the development of new powers under bilateral agreements, generally referred to as International Mutual Legal Assistance Treaties (the other spur being counter-terrorism: Anderson 1989). The association between drugs and money laundering has led to new types of financial policing to 'chase the money' around the international banking system (Dodd-Crompton 1990: 2–8). This opens up a new vista that few would recognise as belonging in the traditional world of policing. In Europe, drug trafficking has been at the forefront of issues of international cooperation through the TREVI group (originally set up to counter terrorism), the so-called 'Schengen' group of countries (France, Germany and the Benelux countries, cooperating to remove border restrictions prior to 1992) and, latterly, the Commission of the European Communities. In Britain, trafficking has stimulated the modernisation of policing, particularly in respect of intelligence and financial investigations, and propelled us half-way towards a national police force (Home Affairs Committee 1990).

Thus, facing the threat of the 'big traffickers', society has taken exceptional measures to safeguard itself. It may therefore seem a contradiction, indeed an insult to common sense, to say that the popular picture of drug trafficking is misleading or even simply wrong. To suggest this is not to imply that every legislative and institutional change that trafficking has provoked or legitimised is a mistake. Measures such as asset confiscation and intelligence development, to be described later in this book, are of considerable potential interest. The judgement upon them depends on how they are used. At this stage, we simply wish to emphasise what a powerful impetus for legislation and organisational change has been provided by the social and political reaction to the prospect of big traffickers, the mafia, drug monopolies, and cartels.

TRAFFICKING MYTHS AND REALITIES

We began this research with no more than a nagging suspicion that, contrary to mythology and media presentation, domestic drug markets might not be organised as neat, top-down hierarchies controlled by a 'Mr Big'.

By the time we were half-way through this research, we were sure of this. At the end, it no longer seems at all remarkable: no cartels; no mafia; no drug barons; and, correspondingly, relatively little corruption – unlike the situation in many plant drug producing countries such as Colombia or Afghanistan. However, when considering such countries, it is important to see that loss or weakness of authority of the central state has been the pre-condition for the emergence of trafficking on a large scale (García Márquez 1990: 91–2; Blok 1974: 10–11).

This distinction – between the social and political conditions in which mass racketeering does and does not emerge – is important to bear in mind, since the exciting images of trafficking that one receives in relation to, say, parts of Latin America can easily get in the way of an understanding of drug markets in Europe. Having made the distinction, we need to admit that some other developed countries, or some regions of such countries, may provide intermediate cases, with Mafia-like or cartel-like features. This may well be the case, for example, in parts of the United States, where patterns of political patronage ('the politics of the pork barrel'), anti-communist machismo and business racketeering go hand in hand (see, for example, the case of Miami: Didion 1987). There, parts of the drug market may take the form of organised crime, intertwined with high-level corruption.

In Britain, however, corruption of the enforcement agencies has been relatively mild, restricted to middle-level scandals involving small groups of officers and low-level 'fit-ups': devastating for those victimised by it, but hardly amounting to the emergence of systematic corruption and the institutionalisation of criminality. European drug markets in general, and British drug markets in particular, exhibit all the features of 'disorganised crime' (cf Reuter 1983), and our research draws out the various forms which the resulting small and medium-scale trafficking can take.

RESEARCHING THE MARKET

The accuracy of any picture based on descriptive research is open to question. It is even more so when the object of research is a group which, by definition, is concealed and invests in secrecy. In the early days of seeking funds for this work we received negative comment on a research proposal because, a referee opined, we had not indicated how we intended to obtain a 'representative' sample of traffickers. This really made us laugh.

Our findings are, of course, influenced by the limited forms of access that we had. Three main routes of access to people who are or were in the past involved in illicit trade in the drug market have been used in the course of the fieldwork on which this book is based. The first was through contact with the enforcement agencies, resulting in interviews with police officers, occasionally with their informants, and focused studies of particularly interesting cases. The second approach was by interviews with people in prisons who have been convicted of drug trafficking offences. Third, key individuals in the community and drug users/traffickers contacted through drug agencies were able to tell us about their own experience, and sometimes put people in touch with us who had been more actively involved in the drug market.

There are, of course, problems inherent in each of these approaches. We gained access to much of our material through enforcement agencies. Here three particular qualifications should be noted. One is that officers were rather keener to tell us about cases which presented them in a reasonable or flattering light.

Second, in some cases we could not be told the whole story since officers had a duty to colleagues or to an informant to withhold certain sensitive information. Third, the informants to whom we were introduced were understandably wary of our role and concerned not to complicate the relationship with their police 'handler'.

We interviewed twenty-five convicted male and female traffickers in prisons. Although imprisoned people are not representative of all criminals (after all, they are untypical in getting caught), our prison interviewees varied markedly in their backgrounds, involvements and declared motivations for talking to us. We think that the variety of perspectives we obtained from our prison interviewees, and their personal experiences of being apprehended, processed, tried and imprisoned make these interviews particularly valuable.

Finally, we interviewed fifty-five people who had in the past been active in the market and, in some cases, heard the story of people's engagement with the enforcement agencies 'from the other side'. Realistically, there are limits to which one can contact traffickers through snowballing without adopting a covert role that would carry dangers and legal complications. We made no attempt to make contact in the way in which an undercover officer or 'participating informant' might (see Chapter 8), preferring to present ourselves as researchers and to accept the limitations of such a role. Nevertheless, we were able to talk at length with a small number of people who were at the time of interview still involved in trafficking in a relatively small way, and a larger number of people who were variously *ex*-traffickers, or 'resting', or had been closely associated with traffickers. The fact that we were open about our interests meant that we could ask direct questions, which would not have been the case if we had been covert participant observers (Burgess 1984: 184–208).

How do you describe something that keeps changing?

As the first interviews were done, we compared our initial impression with the already published literature on drug trafficking, and constructed a typology of drug trafficker/organisations. For a while, this was useful since it served the purpose of a rough sampling grid. We would say, for instance, 'we haven't seen much of that type, do you think it really is that unusual, or are there particular difficulties in finding examples?' We realised that in trafficking cases located by the police, known criminals who turned to trafficking were more common than traffickers with an apparently fully 'legit' background.

There are clear problems with any typology; the world always turns out to be rather more shifting and creative than can be represented as a series of static types. As a starting point, however, we found merit in distinguishing between seven different sorts of trafficking 'firms':

1 *Trading Charities* – enterprises involved in the drug business because of ideological commitments to drugs (e.g. cannabis, Ecstasy), with profit a secondary motive;
2 *Mutual Societies* – friendship networks of user-dealers who support each other and sell or exchange drugs amongst themselves in a reciprocal fashion;
3 *Sideliners* – the licit business enterprise that begins to trade in drugs as a 'sideline';
4 *Criminal Diversifiers* – the existing criminal enterprise that 'diversifies' its operations to include drugs;
5 *Opportunistic Irregulars* – individuals or small groups who get involved in a variety of activities in the 'irregular economy', including drugs;
6 *Retail Specialists* – enterprises with a manager employing people in a variety of specialist roles to distribute drugs to users (an increasingly common 'street dealing' format);
7 *State-sponsored Traders* – enterprises that result from collaboration between control agents and others; for example, collaboration between police undercover agents and their informants who may be allowed to continue to trade; or 'buy bust' covert operations (from Dorn and South 1990).

Now, at the end of the research, we find such a typology less satisfactory, since it cannot represent the fluid picture of the drug market which emerged in greater detail as the fieldwork progressed. As the first four chapters show, evolution of traffickers from one modus operandi to another, partly because of changing pressures from the enforcement side, is quite common. There are also many 'mixed' or difficult to classify cases, such as the alliance between a 'sideliner' who met and married a 'diversifier' (see Chapter 2). Indeed, any attempt to classify social phenomena inevitably does violence to the complexity of what is described, in qualitative as well as quantitative research. Nevertheless, the imposition of some kind of theory, structure or language is inevitable. Few social researchers are naive enough to believe that they can enter the field without preconceptions and that reality declares itself so frankly and directly that no interpretation is necessary (*pace* Glaser and Strauss 1967). We consider it preferable to declare the preconceptions with which we started our research, to see how these preconceptions loosen as the book proceeds.

In the mean time, the typology presented here serves to bring into some kind of focus the diversity of traffickers. Using it as a framework for presenting material on the development of drug markets from the 1960s onwards, we are able to identify some general shifts. In particular, we suggest that there has been a tendency over the past few decades for the more 'amateur' traffickers such as the 'trading charities' to be displaced by more overtly criminal elements. Why this transition to a more professionally criminal and rather more 'heavy' drug market occurred is a much discussed but unanswered question.

RESEARCHING DRUG ENFORCEMENT

We also looked at things from the point of view of law enforcement. Here, we were naturally reliant on enforcement agencies and individuals therein both as a means of general orientation and for specific information. This raised a number of methodological problems, of which the most general is that officers' world-views shaped and limited what they could tell us. Also, as noted previously, officers understandably preferred to tell us about matters which presented them and their squad in a more attractive light. In some cases, we could not be told the whole story since officers had a duty to colleagues or to an informant to withhold certain sensitive information. However, we found that a large number of contacts with officers representing different points of view did provide us with a range of perspectives, some of which had clear resonances with the literature on police work in Britain and the United States.

Part II of the book describes ways in which the enforcement agencies have been responding to trafficking at three levels – national/regional level, county and city police force level, and local level. These levels, it should be made clear, are not stratifications in the drug market – rather, they reflect the organisation of enforcement in Britain. A report from the Association of Chief Police Officers (ACPO) in 1985 (better known as the 'Broome Report') developed this 'three-tier' response. Because this conception has had such a significant impact on the organisation of drug enforcement, we are pleased that ACPO have permitted us to reproduce extracts from it as the Appendix to this book.

The first tier of drug enforcement, national and regional in its scope, consists of a national intelligence unit (combining both police and Customs personnel under Home Office control), together with police Regional Crime Squads. The middle tier is made up by the drug squads of county police forces, city drug squads in major cities, and the Area Drug Squads in London. At the local level, there is some CID (Criminal Investigation Department) and uniformed branch response, targeted at the retail level of the market and at drug users.

We describe some of the enforcement strategies employed by police officers at each of these levels. Chapter 5 describes Regional Crime Squads' operations against traffickers and money laundering. It asks whether enforcement agencies need continuously to change their strategies to frustrate traffickers' attempts to evolve counter-measures. Chapter 6 introduces a city drug squad, then describes an undercover 'buy operation' in which officers offered to purchase drugs in order to bring traffickers out into the open. Chapter 7, on local drug enforcement, includes a description of the recent history of policing in the Notting Hill area of west London, and concludes with a discussion of the US-inspired re-emphasis on 'policing down-market'.

In Part III we look at some of the key issues in drug enforcement for the 1990s. One of the main sources of enforcement activity is the use and cultivation of well-placed informants and in Chapter 8 we look at this sensitive topic. This is an area guarded with secrecy since officers need to protect their informants; it has been the failure to regulate this relationship properly which has led to corruption. In the same chapter we go on to look at 'sell operations', commonly associated with US drug enforcement. There are great sensitivities as to whether or not any sell operations occur in Britain. In a 'sell bust' operation, a police officer or a helpful informant poses as a trafficker and tries to sell drugs to somebody who gets promptly arrested if they oblige. We accept that such operations do not take place in this country. By contrast, in an *extended* sell operation, officers or informants sell drugs not to make an immediate arrest, but as a longer-term intelligence development strategy, gaining information about the market which might otherwise be unobtainable. We suggest that such operations, though officially denied, are being developed in Britain.

A major focus for cooperation between enforcement agencies is the medium of intelligence. In recent years sources of information other than informants have become increasingly important. These include covert operations to develop intelligence, involving buys and possibly sells; financial disclosures from banks and other financial institutions both here and abroad; intelligence about the chemicals used in manufacturing drugs; and public relations campaigns such as the one which orchestrated so much concern about crack cocaine in Europe in 1989 (see Home Affairs Committee 1989a; *Druglink* 1989). Chapter 9 examines how drugs intelligence is developing, both organisationally and operationally, in this complex environment. We show drug trafficking has facilitated the establishment of a National Criminal Intelligence Service (into which the current National Drugs Intelligence Unit will be absorbed) whose capability to direct intelligence development operations make it a *de facto* national detective agency.

MARKETS, CONTROLS AND PENALTIES

This is a book about the control of drug markets and some readers will by now, if not before, be wondering about the underlying aims and assumptions of this study. In particular, there is the question of why bother attempting to control this thing which looks like it is becoming increasingly *un*controllable? Why not instead legalise drugs and settle for state regulation of the market? There are two difficulties with such a proposition and we mention them only briefly. The first is that proponents of legalisation employ a Euro-centric perspective which fails to take account of the impact of legalisation on the economic and social structures of developing countries where plants such as the opium poppy, coca bush and marijuana are grown. Commercialisation would lead to the formation of plantations to rival those of tea, coffee, tobacco, etc. and provide an unsuitable path for development (Dorn 1991). The second difficulty is the pragmatic one that control of trafficking is here to stay, as far as anyone can see into the future. Legalisation of trafficking is simply improbable, given the momentum required to reverse the tide of international agreements (Pearson 1991). We have no objections to a debate about legalisation but such debate does not occur in this book.

In supporting the continuation of prohibition of trafficking we do not associate ourselves with all that is done in its name. We are critical of the upward escalation in imprisonment that characterises most developed countries' response to drug trafficking from the 1960s onwards. Chapter 10 discusses penalties, presenting case studies based upon observation of court cases and interviews with traffickers in prison. One of the inequitable aspects of British drug enforcement is that a naive foreign courier importing one kilo of cocaine may receive a ten-year sentence, whilst a committed British gangster-turned-dealer caught with five times as much (equally potent) amphetamine can receive half that sentence or, quite possibly, be acquitted (cf Chapter 6). The question raised, but not settled here, is whether a criminal justice system that has been designed to inflict exemplary punishments upon major traffickers is taking out its failures on the naive and careless who most easily fall within its grasp. A suspicion that this is the case persists. In respect of the future development of public policy, we suggest that the evolution of financial penalties – from the fine to asset confiscation – together with the development of various kinds of community service, make possible a reversal of expensive and ineffective long prison terms.

These thoughts aside, we have little that we wish to impress upon the reader by way of conclusions. Somewhat against our expectations, we have ended up with a more descriptive study, and a less prescriptive one, than we imagined at the start. In part this is due to greater than expected success in speaking to a broad variety of people on both sides of the legal fence. There is something about this subject that seems to make people want to talk! This is fortunate, since the developments we describe in this book have wide-ranging consequences.

Part I

Drug traffickers

Chapter 1

The good old days
Reciprocity and public service

In Part I we look at drug trafficking individuals and groups as they have evolved in Britain. We take a broadly chronological perspective, looking at the ways in which drug 'dealing' from the 1960s has mutated into drug 'trafficking' in the 1980s/90s. This chapter introduces what some nostalgic interviewees referred to as the good old days, when the supply of drugs was not so much a business, and not as nasty, as it has become.

TRADING CHARITIES

> Dealing was different in those days: no violence, no rip-offs, people actually trusted each other. When you bought or sold, dealer and client invariably sat down and got stoned together – partly sampling the wares but partly social. Nowadays it all seems to be sell and run.
>
> (Harry the cannabis dealer)
>
> All I've ever done is sell to people who want to buy. They have the demand and I have the supply.
>
> (Abby the Ecstasy dealer)

We use the term 'trading charity' to describe those traffickers who, initially at least, are not primarily (and definitely not solely) financially motivated. What financial ambitions they have tend to be thwarted by a lack of business skills and/or by their other, 'social' intentions.

The 1960s hippie passing on cannabis joints to people to turn them on and create peace, love and a better world provides a caricature of this type but, as we show below, this approach to trafficking can be adopted by a quite wide variety of people in differing times. For example, an Australian researcher found this kind of involvement in his study of 'Drug entrepreneurs and dealing culture' in Melbourne in the mid-1970s. This study concluded that dealing in psychedelics had

> moved from a hang-loose ethic linked with the values of the counterculture to a specific attitude which sanctions the accumulation of profit for services rendered.
>
> (Langer 1977: 384)

However, in Langer's research, such dealers rarely made much profit. This, he argued,

> may be partly explained by the fact that entrepreneurial practices related to marketing behaviour have not been entirely coordinated or systematised. . . . For example, there is much waste of their product through constant personal use, gift-giving or entertaining.
>
> (Langer 1977: 384)

Lewis also identifies the significant distinction between those in the drug 'business' as trading charities with a 'hippie' ethic – and those with a more serious profit motive.

> In the late 1960s and early 1970s, many 'hippy' traders and importers dealing in cannabis refused to do business with professional criminals. They did not view themselves as delinquent in an ethical sense and felt threatened by the potential complications of thoroughly criminal connections.
>
> (Lewis 1989: 42)

We now turn to look at some of these individuals and their accounts of who they are prepared to do business with.

Case study: Harry the cannabis dealer

Harry is now in his early forties and was born and has lived for most of his life in a town on the southern coast. He is one of two children and comes from a 'professional' middle-class family. His education was normal and uneventful and with three 'A' levels he entered the local College of Art and Design. Here he quickly became involved in the 'alternative' culture of the 1960s. Looking back he offers the view that this was probably the most exciting period of his life, when friendships and interests were forged which have lasted to date. Drugs, in particular cannabis and LSD, were an important part of this lifestyle. In time, Harry became the 'college dealer', buying cannabis in London and dealing exclusively within his college peer group – he did not regard himself as a 'dealer'.

> I got the money together, hopped on the train to London and scored from any number of contacts in Kensington Market, the Gate [Notting Hill] or the Portobello Road.

Certainly there was no profit motive in this early enterprise,

> I guess I just broke even – my dope was 'free' and it did give me some status. . . . [I was] doing a weight [1 lb. at that time] a week, sometimes more, sometimes less. When I sold out I just went and got more.

In the main, Harry supplied cannabis and he draws attention to the caution which many drug users displayed in the 1960s and which old-style users (whether of cannabis or heroin) today bemoan as frequently absent in a more commercialised and poly-drug using scene:

> Even in those days among us students we did appreciate that some drugs weren't that clever and there was a big distinction between cannabis users and other drug users. I would never deal in speed or anything else although I was sometimes offered it by the guys I was buying from in London. Acid of course was different, I did deal in tabs, mostly from Kensington Market, but when I saw bum trips, I was cautious even of that.

Harry carried on dealing throughout his three years at college, always purchasing in London and dealing in the relatively secure college environment.

> I was never busted but I was careful. We all knew the drug squad officers. Sergeant Bloggs was especially known. He was really out to get the students and used to come to gigs at the college in a Bri-Nylon Beatles wig. It really was like that, cops and robbers stuff, or more like Keystone cops.[2] The people who did get busted were the ones who did crazy things like walk past the police station smoking a joint. Some people almost seemed to want to get busted.

In a familiar move, after completing college, Harry and a group of friends drove a van to Morocco on a camping holiday.

> Of course the real purpose was not camping – it was getting stoned on hash. A last fling before settling down to work and conforming. Anyway, the end result was that we decided to smuggle some hash back. If I'd known the risks involved I'd have never done it. We bought a couple of kilos, it was sand coloured resin with quite a high pollen content, it cost me about £90 but we were so green that I didn't even haggle. Most we hid in sealed packets in the petrol tank, the rest taped inside the spare wheel. There were no problems coming back . . . I dealt it out to a number of friends at really good prices . . . I must have cleared over £250 profit from that one run, which paid for the holiday and left over enough to buy a suit and some shirts for my first job.

However, this period was not to last. After Harry's run to north Africa, he

> went through a period when I was buying on the streets, the odd ounce here and there. However, the drug scene was changing, getting harder and more commercial. People were into dealing for money and that's when things became nasty – once the flower power ethos and era was over. I guess at heart I'm still a hippie, although like most of my contemporaries I look pretty straight. A lot of people got out of drugs then and moved on to other things. It makes me laugh when I look around and work out how many businesses have been established from the profits of one last cannabis run. Really healthy enterprises like [a well known local vegetarian restaurant] and [a silk screen printing outfit].

We shall return to this link between drug trafficking and legitimate business in Chapter 2.

Case study: Abby the Ecstasy dealer

> It seemed that, what with paying for club admission, drinks and everything else, I cleared about £150 a week – not much really. The last couple of runs to town I did make more as he was selling me 100 tablets for £1,000. I spent most of the profit on clothes and records. I know that when I packed it in I had put an extra £200 in my Building Society account.

Abby is a single male in his early twenties. He has lived all his life in his home town, attended a local comprehensive school, then worked in a bank and then a fashion store. He lived for two years with Andy and now shares a house with three other gay men and works in a record shop. He started to use Ecstasy and a few other drugs as part of his involvement in the club scene.

When I met Andy we were both very much into the local club scene but at that time, late 1986, there wasn't that much drugs around, at least in the sort of clubs we went to. Some cannabis, poppers – but mostly booze. AIDS was becoming high profile and most young gay men were into a health kick, body image was important, one didn't want to look ill, so everyone was into gyms and sunbeds. I used a little cannabis which Andy didn't like too much and that was it.

What changed Abby's involvement was the link in the clubs between Acid House music and dancing and Ecstasy.

I was at the time going up to the West End clubs in London – and the one where Acid House started in the UK. It was originally a gay thing, a split off from energy dancing. It was there that I had my first Ecstasy tab, 1987. From then I was going up every weekend for allnighters. This was long before it had become a straight music and the *Sun* [newspaper] got involved. Everyone says Ecstasy is bad; however, when it was confined to the gay scene there didn't seem to be any problems at all. People just took it and had a good time. They were all tightly interlinked, the clubs you went to, what one wore, the music one listened to and taking Ecstasy. At that time without the press involved it was discreet and very much a closed group doing it in very specific environments. I was going to the clubs all the time and got to know a lot of people so when Acid House came to the local club scene, I was in from the start.

When asked about how he became involved in 'dealing' Ecstasy, Abby's immediate reaction was a dismissal of the term 'dealing'.

I don't like that word. It pictures a stereotype who is making money from others' misfortune. Ecstasy, at least initially, wasn't like that. When Acid House started locally, it did actually change things. Up until then, gays went to one sort of club and straights to another; there was no mixing, unless you count 'queer bashing' as such. [Then] Acid House led to a new club scene, young gays and straights in the same clubs without problems, since they were both there for the same reason – the music. It's a bit like reggae, that brought together young blacks and skinheads with a common interest – music and cannabis. Ecstasy was – and here I do agree with the newspapers – essential to Acid House, everyone wanted to take Ecstasy. The group with the experience and who could get the drug were young gay men. So I got into supplying simply because I knew the contacts in London from my time spent up there at gay discos. It was quite easy.

With everything so easy and so pleasant, Abby explored the prospects for getting larger deals.

As I said, I had been buying in the London discos for nearly a year, most weekend nights, always from the same guy. It was always quite open in there [in a particular club], everyone knew him, you just went across and bought. I spoke to the man I had always bought from in London. . . . He told me – and I would emphasise that he did know me, I'd bought from him at least forty times – that he could sell me fifty tabs for £600. That's just over £10 each and they sell from £16 to £20 each. I withdrew almost all my savings from the Building Society – I had been saving for a holiday. I should say that he gave me a number to ring when I had the money. It was a portaphone and he arranged to meet me at a pub in Swiss Cottage. . . . Anyway, I turned up sweating but he was there with another man. They didn't have the tablets with them but asked for the money. I felt that he was hardly likely to cheat, since he was in the club every night so it's not as if I couldn't find him. Anyway, they took the money and went off. I was told to wait in the Underground station. After about half an hour, this second man came into the station and told me to buy a ticket to Baker Street. We got on the train together and he gave me the tablets during the journey. He got off at Baker Street and I saw him going across to catch a northbound train so I think they always used the underground for passing across bulk shipments. I bought from him about six times – at the end I was buying 100 tablets at a time and the method was always the same. Telephone him, go up on the train, meet him in the pub and pass across the money. Then be given the tablets at the Underground station. After the first time they didn't pass the tablets across on the train, but on the platform as I was waiting for the train. It seemed to be a different person each time who passed across the tablets.

In Abby's view this procedure was a secure one and he felt that added safety derived from these contacts also being gay.

They were all gay – sorry, I should have said that at the beginning. I think it's much better buying from someone who's the same as you. That's safer. . . . I think that they must have been shifting a lot of tablets – they never had any problems in supplying me and the tablets were always the same – white with a groove. There's not that much [more] to tell. I went to the local club with my tablets. At that time people were asking each other who had got and who sold Ecstasy. There was no trouble in getting rid of them. I'd pick up from London early on a Friday evening and be back in town by 8.30 p.m. Some I would sell that night and the remainder on the Saturday night. Most customers wanted one or two, but occasionally people would want more, say five if they were buying for friends as well. I used to leave most of the tablets with a friend and pick up from him when I needed more and also give him the money to hold. He was happy with £30 and a couple of free tablets for an evening.

Abby stopped supplying Ecstasy as he became disenchanted with the Acid House disco scene – ruined by a bad press and being taken up by

different people, real lager louts and 'loadsamoney'. They weren't in it for the music or dancing, just there since the papers said it was deviant and they thought it was trendy. . . . When it grew people saw a chance to make a lot of money – clothing, records, clubs and drugs. Most of the Ecstasy around in town now is a load of rubbish and that's why you see so many bad reactions – Acid and Speed mixed together and sold in capsules for a fortune. . . . Once the entertainment industry saw that there was money to be made, Acid House died – and it's the same with any music, once it's taken up for profit there's a lot lost.

Even given the recent nature of Acid House as a music form, it has passed and Abby's account of his association with a particular drug that was homologous (fitted into) to the culture (cf Willis 1978) is already full of nostalgia and regret at the commercialisation and betrayal of the Acid House scene. He now goes to a number of different London clubs, no longer comfortable with the image that the local venues project and, perhaps more significantly, he no longer deals (or 'supplies') any drugs at all.

In the USA, the West Coast ex-hippie dealers and smugglers in Adler's (1985) study represent a similar picture of the trading charity. The size and scale of their operations may become significant for a while, but their profits are diminished and their involvement often curtailed by 'a residual hedonistic "hippy" ideology' (Lewis 1989: 37; Adler 1985).

The Trading Charity dealer ties involvement in the supply of drugs to a particular facet of their social life and *socialising* within it. This may not amount to a full-blown ideology or world-view but it does mean that a goal of profit accumulation is subsidiary to, or strongly tempered by, a commitment to or enjoyment of the social and cultural aspects of using the drug and the context in which this is done. Such considerations are shared to some extent by the next type of trafficking network to be described.

MUTUAL SOCIETIES: RECIPROCAL SUPPLIERS

A mutual society is a friendship or acquaintance-based network of drug users, some of whom, some of the time, will supply drugs to others. Reciprocity is the name of the game (Auld 1981) – every user is potentially a supplier, and everyone is expected to help out everyone else. It is in this respect that they are *unlike* the trading charity dealers discussed above, since the latter supply their own needs from their trading stock, rather than trailing round their customers and trying to 'score' from them.

Members of mutual societies, or user-dealers as they are sometimes called, constitute a large population in relation to other types of traffickers. Where they have made links to helping agencies such user-dealers have been the group most easily, and hence most frequently, researched in studies of drug dealing and drug markets.

At one point going back about eight years we met as a group . . . I mean all of us together . . . we knew each other and it was sort of like a club thing you know, it's not as if there were membership cards or anything like that, but it was just a very isolated little group as such . . . and if gear wasn't so easy to find so you know you kept it within your group. . . . I mean at one point if you didn't have any money one day you could go to a friend and say 'well lend me a quarter and I'll pay you back tomorrow' sort of thing. But now you can't do that – people are very money oriented, there's always a risk because there are so many more people using it.

(Mick)

As we can see at the end of Mick's account, those who were involved in reciprocal networks lapse easily into nostalgia, most often expressed as a sense of sadness at the way in which the market has changed.

I think there's this profit thing has changed the dealing sort of side as well so there's a lot of changes that seemed to have happened, there doesn't seem to have been very clear how it happened or why it happened.

(Chris)

At first glance, the mutual society seems to be most closely linked to the use and trade of cannabis rather than 'harder' drugs. Johnson's (1980: 116) 'cannabis subculture', for instance, seems to fit this well.

The cannabis subculture promotes the sharing of marijuana and hashish. A joint is frequently shared by many at a party or where a peer group congregates. Usually, no money is involved in such sharing but different group members are expected to provide the drug at various times. Distribution norms expect weekly or more frequent users to buy their own supply and/or to share with others.

However, as is well known, mutual societies certainly do not confine themselves to cannabis (Fraser and George 1988). Research done in the north-west of England by Parker *et al.* suggested that the norms of sharing that originally developed around cannabis were for some people quite easily extended to another drug that might be smoked/inhaled, heroin, when that became quite widely available. As one of their respondents said

> We just used to hang around with each other and it was one
> of those things, like, you'd never done before. We got into
> pot at the same time, we got into acid at the same time and
> then there was more smack around than pot, so we got into
> that.
>
> (Parker *et al.* 1988: 48)

Parker *et al.* describe such transitions as an effect of 'peer group
pressure'. This involves both conformity to what had become the
group's norm and the threat of possible exclusion if one failed to
conform. The networking of drug users and user-dealers forms a
social and economic world built around scoring and using drugs.
In this situation, dealing helps to maintain the pattern of usage.
There is a marked absence of any professional sense of drug
selling.

Something of the amateurishness of user-dealers is confirmed by
one of Pearson's (1987: 122) respondents laughingly recounting his
first attempt at dealing.

> I tried to sell it once. . . . [But as it ended up] I just took it . . .
> instead of selling it! You know, me and this lad went halves and
> bought two grams, and then he got arrested. So I just chased
> [smoked] it all . . .

Another sense of the different ethic which characterises mutuality
is provided by Mick's account of selling.

> It seems no matter how much gear you have each day, say I was
> given two grams to get rid of in a day, you never seemed to
> make a profit . . . in the papers they say that you know people
> that are using gear are doing it primarily for profit. [But] I mean
> if you are using gear you can kiss the profit goodbye, there is
> no profit because the funny thing with heroin is that the more
> gear you get the more you sell the more you use. You use up
> the profit.
>
> (Mick)

A similar sentiment pervades Stewart's description of some sellers.

> When they first start selling gear and are operating from
> home, dealers begin by inviting their customers in. Everyone
> sits around chatting and taking drugs in a relaxed friendly
> atmosphere.
>
> (Stewart 1987: 119)

New and inexperienced users can enter into a network of usage and dealing based simply on the pragmatic aspects of scoring.

If you are a new user you will probably score at the lowest level of the junk pyramid, buying small bits now and again from a personal friend. He will be unlikely to be well known to the police because he is not, in any formal sense, a regular dealer. . . . Whether you live in a tower block or a stately home, your own little scene fosters and feeds your habit. This scene might include anything from ten to a hundred interdependent users who form a secret network where people can mix and mingle, with the underlying aim of buying, selling and consuming drugs.

(Stewart 1987: 37)

Similarly in Fagan's (1989) typology of youth gangs with drug involvements, 'party gangs' are described.

Their drug sales, in the absence of other forms of crime, are likely to be supportive of their own drug use. Their extensive involvement in drug use suggests that their affiliation may be based on mutually supportive patterns of drug use and dealing to support group and individual drug use. This type seems to be a 'party gang' that otherwise manifests several of the subcultural and organisational features of gangs.

(Fagan 1989: 649–50)

Such users operate as a loose network, with a commonality of interest, on the street. For example, Agar (1978: 260) describes the response to a heroin shortage in which, 'The addict group turned inward and exchanged information relevant to the search for an alternative supply of narcotics'. Similarly Moore (1977: 47–51) points out that users can have difficulty in finding out the prices and locations of heroin sales. One response is that users exchange relevant information about 'market conditions', such as the best places, people, times to buy, reasonable prices and so on (see Stewart 1987: 121). The advantages of 'keeping in contact' in this way can again be related to the pragmatic aspects of obtaining one's supply of drugs.

The more users and dealers you know, the better your chance of keeping yourself supplied. Remaining aloof means trouble; it means not knowing where else to go when your regular dealer hits a bad patch or gets arrested. In every small group

of interdependent users, there is always someone with a foot
in another camp. In that camp there will be others with contact
elsewhere.

(Stewart 1987: 63)

Two long-term drug users talked to us about the way in which they
and their acquaintances used to support their own consumption in
a way that randomised benefits around the group. Sarah and Pete,
involved in long-term heavy-drug use in and around Metroplace
since the late 1960s, described a more whimsical, 'pot luck' example
of dealing in stolen pharmaceutical drugs among social contacts.
Within the network that they knew in the late 1960s, there was
held to be a 'regular price' for a stolen pharmacist's chest and a
chest might be stolen and sold very quickly, without being opened
– or at least that is the contention. 'Sometimes it would contain
drugs that made it a bargain and other times you'd be less lucky.'
As time went on, however, and more people got involved, a more
hard-headed approach began to prevail and the cabinet would
be opened, its contents identified and then the different drugs
would be sold to different dealers who had different markets.
This reflects a diversity of markets and participants based upon
divisions between local drug using subcultures, with 'the hippies
into cannabis; the black clubs and shebeens also selling cannabis;
the speed freaks and the junkies'. Exposure in all these different
groupings does, of course, inevitably increase one's vulnerability
to police action and hence dealers at this point are likely either
to take on more business to make their risk worthwhile, or else
to retreat back into the relative security of the mutual society or
trading charity role. It was this latter course that Sarah and Pete
followed, fearing any involvement with either the police or heavy
dealers, and turning instead to paying for their own heroin with
income from the sale of the house left to Pete by his parents.

The norm of reciprocity underpinning the exchange of drugs and
information about their supply can operate over the short, medium
or long term. Very few drug users seem to operate a strict rule of
reciprocity in the way that many drinkers in the public house will
adhere to the 'round' system of taking turns to buy. The typical
user-dealer seems to reciprocate over the medium term, or at least
to attempt to do so, or to construct an appearance of doing so, in
order to 'keep in' with his or her group. In some cases, however, the
reciprocity will be looser and articulated over a much longer-term

period – years rather than weeks. The early drug-using history of Hugh provides a personal account of how, during the 1960s, people who were interested in sharing drugs would take turns in obtaining them. For Hugh – who is now serving a sentence of eight years for the attempted smuggling of a large consignment of cannabis – the attraction of the drug scene was its social network, with money a secondary concern.

> It was a cult, it was most certainly a cult . . . lots and lots of upper-middle-class and upper-class people, it was a mixing of the classes if you like, it broke down class barriers at the time. . . . They were all working people, all smoked at weekends – they're not killing their babies, they're very nice sensible people, in fact I'm the only criminal among them. . . . Dental technicians, doctors, building workers, dockers, there really isn't a vocation not there. . . . You're talking about people in the hippie days, someone would go to India and bring back a kilo, another would bring back a kilo from somewhere else . . . at that time it was 90% like that. [It was] before there were 'animals' [profit-oriented dealers]. . . It was a very stable pattern, people who'd gone for three months' holiday and when they came back they brought some hashish with them, be it three ounces or two kilos. . . . From 1965 to 1973 . . . it went from £8 to £10 [for an ounce of hashish].

As Hugh goes on to describe, those days were numbered.

> In 1973 it started going up very fast from ten to twelve to fifteen to twenty-five to thirty to forty – it kept going up. It then reached a peak of £80 an ounce and then the big boys came in. . . . We've put all this in the hands of very, very irresponsible people and all they care about is how much [money they can make].

A final comment on the collapse of any sense that drug trafficking could be a reciprocal affair or motivated by ideas of public service is given by Jane, a former user-dealer. Asked about the idea of mutual societies she said, 'That went years ago. It's like dog eat dog'. It is to the question of how drug traffickers adapted to this bracing new climate that we now turn.

Chapter 2

Going for cover
Trafficking as a sideline

As British drug markets have developed and become established, so the dynamics of the market and trends in law enforcement have tended to push out those who, like the trading charities we discussed in the preceding chapter, were making those markets for reasons that were more 'social' than financial.

To take the cannabis market, for example, it is clear that increased policing made trafficking more dangerous, leading to many dealers feeling that the risk was no longer worth the slim financial margins that many were working on. At the same time, more 'money-minded' people, with serious business sense and financial ambitions got involved. There were three choices facing the trading charity – get out; get some kind of legal business cover to facilitate and disguise the drug dealing; or get involved with the more serious and competent criminals coming into the drug trade.

Quite a few took the first option, temporarily or permanently, and quit dealing. Some, like Harry the cannabis dealer introduced in chapter 1, took the middle option, as we shall shortly describe. They developed a licit business 'cover' for their drug business. Finally, a few took the third option, and stayed in the drug business, developing a cautious and sometimes rather frightened relationship with some of the more experienced criminal types who were seeing opportunities in drugs.

This chapter and Chapter 3 then, are about two 'career options' for drug traffickers that developed from the 1970s onwards: going for the cover of a legitimate business, and getting more involved in the criminal underworld. In relation to drug markets that have only relatively recently developed, such as the Ecstasy market of the late 1980s, trading charities were initially able to operate with relatively little pressure from the police or major criminals, largely because usage and selling took place within relatively insulated subcultures. But as that market matured, the same pressures became apparent there, too – as the case study of Abby in Chapter 1 illustrates. It seems that only in the early stages of a drug scene can drug trafficking be a casual affair.

SIDELINERS: THE COVER OF A LEGITIMATE BUSINESS

Harry, introduced in Chapter 1, discontinued his cannabis dealing (and much of his cannabis consumption) because of the increasing commercialisation of the drug scene, and because it began to get 'nasty'. Family considerations also played a part. He spent the next twelve years developing a career and raising a family and indicated that most of his friends were doing the same. His cannabis use was minimal and generally confined to visits with old friends. Then, in the early 1980s he and his wife established a business which provided an opportunity to re-create his trading charity, even in the chillier conditions of the 1980s.

> The company is quite successful and I employ several people. As part of my job I go across once a week to Holland. . . . It's a regular run and I use the same ferry. The whole drug scene in Holland is much easier – dope [cannabis] is practically legal, so I started buying small amounts and using again on a regular basis. An old college friend of mine, Alex, now works in Amsterdam and in the advertising business. I know he's run some fair quantities of dope across to England in the exhibition stands that his company uses, and he comes over to set them up. He introduced me to a guy who's a big dealer, he's Dutch and he can supply virtually anything – Leb., Pak., Moroccan, even genuine Afghanistan black which I haven't seen for years – the stuff that's alleged to be pressed down with camel piss – you can see the salt crystals in it from the piss. . . . Apparently, you do have to be careful in Holland 'cause there is a whole industry packing and pressing low-quality dope into something that looks top grade – especially for the English trade. So Alex's introduction was a real help. I think what I also liked is that this Dutch guy seemed like a time-warped English hippie – the way he dressed and the music he listened to.

To us, Harry's contact sounds rather like an undercover police officer, but he offered Harry the sense of security he needed to get back into the drug market on the terms that first attracted him.

> I paid cash £750 for the half kilo and when I got home was able to knock out ounces at £80, which isn't bad for top-grade Leb. This gave a profit of about £500 but I think I must have smoked most of it. I'm not greedy, I just bring back half a kilo a month on average and just sell to friends and never in less than weighed ounces. It's a service, not a profit business so it helps us all.

Harry is confident about the security that protects these transactions. The chances of a customer passing information to the police is, he thinks, low since he continues his 1960s guideline of supplying only to friends. His legitimate business gives him an opportunity to get the supplies he needs. And he is confident that, if he did get into trouble, his friends and customers would rally round.

> I guess I'm doing what I did in the '60s, for the same reasons. Things have just changed and got up to date. Although it's still the same – a service for friends, if I was in trouble with my business or whatever they'd all help me. We all go back a long way.

Harry's story shows one of the ways in which a legitimate business can 'sideline' in drug trafficking. There are, as we will see, a number of variations on this theme. What these cases have in common is an existing legitimate business to use as a base. It may have premises, transport and other resources useful for drug distribution activities; it may or may not be facing or anticipating adverse trading conditions; it has or can acquire capital for investment; and it has the flexibility to take up opportunities for investment without too much difficulty. Participation in the drug market is a risk-venture, a considered gamble judged to have a sufficiently attractive pay-off. As such it is infrequent and may be a one-off occurrence.

In the following account offered by Dick and Carla, two ex-user-dealers from north London, a friend of theirs moved from starting out with a (relatively) legitimate business, through being a serious 'fence', to dealing in cocaine.

> Carla: There is a friend of mine . . . [and] all the young people who are on heroin who are thieves, stealing tellies, videos, jewellery, will take it to this person and he will buy it off them. . . .

Q. How did he start out?

Dick: He was a legitimate antiques dealer. His son got into
drugs and I suppose his son took him into it.

Carla: No, hold on, to start off he was a legitimate antiques
dealer and then, you know, antique dealers, most of
them, in their own little way, are bent, y'know, to get
their bargains.

Dick: They've got their 'ducks and dives'.

Carla: He started, instead of just buying antiques off the thieves,
he started buying electrical goods as well which was
making him a lot of money, so that was his next thing
[i.e. developing as a fence]

Dick: Say, you've got a video, if you're desperate you'll sell that
for £50, he'll sell it for £200.

Carla: You know, you walk in the house and he's got tellies
stacked up. . . . He found another good way of making
money was in cocaine. His son was selling it and he took
it over from his son.

One occupation apparently at high risk in this regard is being a
publican. Examples were provided in several interviews. Dick
offers this recollection:

I used to drink in this pub all the time. There used to be a crowd
of us and they were all villains who I used to drink with. I was
only accepted amongst them because a member of my family
was a friend of all of them. I was only young, about nineteen,
twenty. [Dick is now twenty-six.] I remember one night, I heard
a bloke talking and he said he was ten grand short for a shipment
of puff [cannabis]. And he [the publican] said 'I'll lay out the
ten grand. What do I get back for it?' And he [other] said
'you get fifteen grand back'. And he [publican] said, 'when?'
And he [other] said, 'within a week'. And like I presume it
took place because they were doing deals often together [after
that].

We have heard many similar stories about publicans. Here is
Frank, a police informant, describing pubs as venues for large-scale
dealing.

Criminal fraternities or gangs would have territory and their
territory would be modified to help the sale of drugs. Like
discotheques would be introduced, loud music, bright lights,

different kinds of facilities would be introduced to cater for the drug user. Like there's one particular pub . . . you can stand there and something like £100,000 will change hands. [There would be] £5,000 to £10,000 deals going on, you know, ten or twenty times a day. There's wholesale pubs and there's retail pubs.

Derek, an ex-user from Valleytown, Wales, was impressed by the sideliners he had met in prison.

My friend in jail, as I say, he is quite an eminent professional person. He sold out as a faster way of making money and he's got several houses, owns a big chunk of land in one of the towns in Wales. You know, it paid. It paid him, under the cover of being a building firm he managed to account for his apparent wealth. His two co-accused as well – there's three guys – [and] you'd never imagine that they were the kind of people that would go into the smuggling of cannabis by the ton.

Another illustration of the sideliner is the case of Michael, a European in his mid-forties. Michael had a stake in several gambling clubs and had been involved in this business since the late 1970s, although his interest in gambling was long-standing. He had previously worked in the travel business and had organised trips to fly players to casinos. His family was established in the antiques trade, so Michael's background was firmly in the world of the small but profitable – and generally speaking, wholly legitimate – business. Acting as a freelance agent, he developed a role as a person who could perform useful introductions, make links and bring together people who shared mutual business interests. In this capacity he actively sought out developing business deals where he could perform this function. He says that he even did some work for Imelda Marcos of the Philippines when he heard that she was interested in a particular work of art. Surprisingly, or perhaps just naively, he says that all of these movements and connections did not look suspicious at all until they were examined in terms of possibly being related to drug trafficking. His involvement in the latter, he claims, 'was a mistake', very limited and something he 'didn't need'. Michael says that all he had done was to extend his role as a go-between and contact-person into the drug business in a limited way by bringing together a group of people with a mutual interest in importing cannabis from the Netherlands into Britain. This was the extent of his involvement, he says, and he was reluctant to say too much about the sellers and buyers. The buyers, based in the UK, were themselves involved in licit business.

> In the past they had nothing to do with drugs, but they obviously realised there was some financial benefit and they knew some people [whom they could work with to supply].

The contact-making and business life that he had previously been involved in looked very suspicious under the glare of a police investigation. Michael received a sentence of ten years.

Trafficking as a sideline to prostitution

In Britain, prostitution is not in itself illegal, though it is considered 'shady' and surrounded with legal restrictions. It is a form of business that offers opportunities for drug trafficking to the prostitute's clients.

In 1988, Jill, a prostitute, was sentenced to fifteen years for conspiracy to supply heroin and also supplying persons unknown (which on appeal was reduced to nine years). The only drugs found in her possession was approximately one ounce of heroin, but there was damaging evidence from a pager, and the jury and judge accepted prosecution inferences of dealing small amounts over a long period.

Jill describes her background as a resident of west London who has three main sources of income: buying and selling houses with the father of her child; prostitution (and it was in connection with this that she used her pager, she says); and supplying drugs in the limited sense of being a user-dealer who would sometimes be buying and sometimes selling. Previously she worked as a beautician. She has four children and says 'I'm a single mother and have to make money for my family'.

Of the circumstances surrounding her arrest she says:

> I saw Tony [a person of broadly similar background] in August 1987 and didn't see him again until September when he came to my flat. I later found out that the police had been following him. He didn't come into my flat but drove around the block with his wife and children. He then waited for fifteen minutes

in the pub car park. Then he came into my flat and I got twenty quid's worth of heroin off him. After that the police continued to follow him but lost him for forty minutes. Then they jumped on him and arrested him and in his home they found several ounces of speed in a sock. That evening the police came to my house at five to twelve and there was obviously nothing there [she had taken or sold the heroin she had bought] so they left.

Then in October the Portsmouth police came to my house with a warrant for my arrest. I was refused bail and was put up as Tony's main supplier – even though they knew that I was not supplying him that day because they had trailed him to Bethnal Green and only found five grammes of speed which his wife had in her pocket. The conspiracy was supposed to work in the sense that I was the only one with money, so I must have been the supplier.

At committal, Jill faced six charges of conspiracy, all very similar charges but with slight variations in the lists of names of those alleged to have conspired. There were altogether eighteen charges on the indictment, of which six referred to her in one way or another.

Of the ten persons charged, one had fled to Spain, seven pleaded guilty, and she and one other pleaded not guilty. It was a legal aid case, since all Jill's assets were frozen.

They took out an injunction to freeze my bank account and my shares and to stop me selling my car so it had to be legal aid.

Legal representation was not very stable and her original barrister was replaced the afternoon before the trial by two others from the same firm. On the morning of the trial, the defence side received an 'offer' from the prosecution.

The offer was five years and [asset] confiscation of £18,000 if I would go guilty.

However, she persisted with a not guilty plea, partly because – she maintains – she was not guilty as charged. She does not deny that she is a habitual criminal.

I've been taking drugs and dealing drugs and been arrested for drugs and had two prison sentences before.

But she does claim that (a) she was not dealing to the extent alleged by the prosecution and (b) that some of her transactions were in relation to cocaine, not heroin (the only drug mentioned in the charges). Why, then, does she think that she was found guilty and sentenced so severely? She gives several reasons.

> On the grounds that I had money, that's what it comes down to. The other nine people in the case, they were cleverer than me, and they don't open bank accounts.

Second, the prosecution argued that the pager showed evidence of dealing to a number of people over a long period. The pager evidence seems to have been very damaging, though Jill says that only some of it truly refers to the drug named in the charges, heroin.

> I had a pager system that I used for prostitution as well as drugs and there would be messages like 'Pop over to Tony's for a port and lemon'. They made that out to mean that I should go to Portsmouth in connection with a load of heroin. But some of it was about prostitution and some about cocaine.

Jill maintains that some of the numbers on the pager referred to cocaine, not heroin. Furthermore, there were notes in her house clearly relating to cocaine transactions. However, she says, the police were not in this case attempting to prove a cocaine conspiracy, so this potential evidence was ignored. All the numbers were taken to refer to heroin.

> The police disregarded the notes on top of the freezer with references to coke, they left that behind because they weren't looking for a cocaine user or dealer. The judge said to the jury, in view of the charges, if you believe that she had been dealing in cocaine, then you must find her not guilty.

However, she was found guilty on the charges of conspiring to supply and supplying persons unknown. In sentencing, the judge accepted prosecution suggestions that the numbers on the pager amounted to supplying a total of six kilograms of heroin in small lots in less than six months. He then said that he believed that she had been active over a period twice as long, and so doubled the total amount to twelve kilogrammes, estimated street value £2 million. He gave her fifteen years for conspiring to supply. Additionally he ordered £30,000 asset confiscation. (Jill had £18,000 in the bank, £8,000 in stocks and shares, a £3,000 car, £700 in cash and £600 in travellers' cheques.) She appealed and her sentence was reduced to nine years.

Jill's case shows some of the advantages and disadvantages of 'sidelining' in drugs from an established and legal business base – a mixture of prostitution and buying and selling houses, in the case of Jill and the father of her child. The positive side is that the business may offer opportunities for trafficking and for concealing that trafficking. The downside is that, if one is caught and convicted, the financial and other evidence of long-term trafficking can get one a heavy sentence.

'Dipping in and out of dealing'

People who use a legitimate business enterprise – or their employment within such an enterprise – as a base for drug trafficking are quite often aware of the danger that they are likely to lose both legitimate and illegitimate sources of income if they operate too flagrantly. A common response to this worry is to deal in drugs for short periods only.

Cliff's story illustrates such a pattern. Cliff left school at sixteen with no qualifications but through his dad he became apprenticed to a plumber.

> However, I blew that as I wasn't very interested in plumbing and then drifted into a whole range of dead-end jobs.

Cliff moved from job to job and, as family relations deteriorated, moved out of the family home and into 'a house of bedsits that was a bit of a pit'. The cheap rent, however, left him with more disposable income from whatever job he was doing. He had tried cannabis and speed before but now mixed in a world where

> Everyone . . . was using [heroin] at that time [around 1970] and I worked hard to become a junkie. The pattern from then on was predictable, working lost its attraction, I got into thieving or any other villainy that was around. I got caught a number of times for minor offences – shoplifting, social security fraud, cheque fraud, possession of stolen property – nothing particularly heavy, no custodial sentences, just fines and probation.

Cliff went through a bad spell in which his heroin habit grew and so did his involvement in petty crime. He was not dealing in drugs at this time but was 'either hassling for money or hanging out or trying to hit doctors or buy codeine linctus'. He moved to a different town but continued using heroin and 'thieving' to pay for it. After a two-year prison sentence and a subsequent six-month stay at a rehabilitation house imposed by a court for a different offence, he settled down in a steady personal relationship, stopped using and had a 'regular job working on the taxis'. When the relationship broke up, Cliff returned to his home town and by 1986 had started working on the taxis there. He discovered that many of the drivers were snorting speed 'as a way of keeping going during the night shifts'. Cliff started using himself and 'almost by accident' he says, 'became the company dealer'.

> I used to go across to someone I knew on an estate and buy an ounce every day for cash. This guy would only deal in cash. . . . It wasn't the best speed in the world but it wasn't rubbish and he always had it available, so there was never any running around from dealer to dealer trying to score. . . . Dealing was easy because everyone just called me up on the radio and I arranged our cabs would meet somewhere. It was very safe, everyone paid in cash – as taxi drivers they all carried quite a lot of money and there were plenty of chances of fiddling on the job.

Success bred unwanted fame.

> Of course, a good system like that did not stay quiet for long. People began to know I was dealing and got to know my cab number. People used to call up the taxi office and 'book a cab' and ask for my cab number. When I got round they wanted to score some speed. So I did some business that way, however I wasn't too happy about that because once you get known as a dealer then when someone does get busted they are singing your name all over the place in the hope of getting off lightly from the police. . . . Also when people are informing the police they tend to say you're a much bigger dealer than you are because that looks better for them than merely informing on someone who's just splitting up one gramme a day.
>
> I must have been making £500 a week profit from the speed business and after about six months I decided to get out. I didn't want to push my luck and anyway I was becoming a nervous

wreck – getting paranoid and using too much speed didn't help. I don't think people realise what a lot of strain there is on a dealer, it's not easy profit, it's hard-earned money. That's why people tend to dip in and out of dealing . . . you're heading for a heart attack if you don't rest.

Even in the irregular economy it would seem, at least according to this respondent, the stress and tension of work-life threaten 'burn-out'. In this, as in other matters – and whatever the morality of the claims – participation in the workings of the drug market seems to mirror activity in legitimate business. And, as both this and the next and final case study in this chapter show, the legitimate and illegitimate worlds interact.

Case study: the interaction between legitimate business and established criminals

One of the most important aspects of the involvement of originally legitimate businesses in the drug market is the provision not simply of 'cover' for travel and trade, but also of a means of laundering the money involved.

In this case study of the sometimes close linkage between a business sideliner and an established criminal (a type whose increasing involvement in the drug trade from the 1970s onwards is described more fully in the next chapter), we describe a husband and wife team of unrepentant traffickers. They see cannabis as not very harmful and justify their involvement in its trafficking by reference to the over-taxation of the legitimate economy. They were arrested with over 200 kilos of cannabis with two couriers who had been hired for the job. They were initially charged with importation, but the charges were subsequently changed to conspiracy to import cannabis on ten occasions. They were convicted in 1989 and sentenced to ten years for the husband, seven years for the wife, and five and six years respectively for the two couriers. The wife was pregnant on her arrest and, when she realised how long the remand period was likely to be, had an abortion in prison.

She is Belgian and he is American. Her background is that her parents were divorced when she was ten years old and she then lived with her mother. Her father was a building contractor and her mother a real estate agent. She admits to turning into a 'difficult teenager', married early and then divorced. Family money allowed her to start up a bar which she ran for several years, before her first husband undermined the business. She started all over again by studying public relations, then worked on several right-wing political campaigns.

> The government must support those with money, middle-class people and big companies, who if they have to pay a lot of tax will not be able to flourish. I blame high tax rates for many problems. When I had my bar sometimes I ended up with less money than the people working for me. Our European countries are over-socialised. The spirit used to be 'what can I do for my country?'; nowadays it's 'what can my country do for me?'

It was whilst moving in these circles that she met her second husband-to-be.

> We went horse-riding and played tennis, we got along fine. At that time I thought he was a businessman. As soon as he found out that my [moral] principles were lax, he said that I could go along with his view of things, or not.

Unbeknown to her at that stage, the husband had previously been arrested for conspiracy to defraud an insurance company for several hundred thousand pounds. More recently he had specialised in cannabis trading.

> He used other people to get it out of Morocco, Spain or whatever. When we were arrested we were only dealing with one set of people. Somebody grassed us up – perhaps because my husband was getting too big.

They were incriminated by one of their couriers, who had been persuaded by Customs to provide information.

> We were in a hotel [in England] and we were meant to meet the courier to take the drugs, and my husband and I got arrested. Because I was a foreigner I pretended to have no English. They told me I was arrested and told me my rights, then started asking questions. . . . Questioning for me was easy because they felt that I was not involved. Then they thought that I had information and started putting pressure on me. What they wanted me to do was to grass my husband but they never offered me a deal and my solicitor advised me against it anyway.

Their defence in court was that

> The whole case was 'iffy' because John said that he wasn't involved in the drugs smuggling, he was only involved in the laundering. . . . [And] I said that I was coming over to England and I was involved in opening up my new art gallery [in Belgium] and had my connections [in England] but I was too busy to notice what my husband was doing. We were cross-examined for three days. We showed papers for cars we had bought and sold.

Whilst there was a variety of bits of evidence that contributed to the verdicts of guilty, it was the pattern of previous trips together that seemed decisive.

> The conspiracy charge was from August 1987 until August 1988 and in that time in we made ten trips. That's how they do it!

Also, the wife alleged, British Customs falsified evidence.

> In the investigation they [Customs] tried to falsify evidence. There was no evidence to connect us with the second car [the couriers', which carried the drugs]. They sealed up evidence from our private car and six months later, a bag of our property that came from nowhere got into that car. What I believed happened in those six months is that they realised that the courier was not going to talk in court, so they were afraid that we were going to walk. But we were able to cast reasonable doubt on the bag in the Merc.

Be that as it may, the wife's account of her part in the money laundering is of considerable interest. First, a series of false business receipts would be prepared, showing 'legitimate' income covering the income expected to be derived from the drugs.

> It all worked with false bills, false receipts. For example, what went through my legitimate business was money for film extras and so on and it is quite easy in Belgium you don't need to declare tax on such a business. And the reason I went into the art business is that it is even more easy, buying and selling pictures. It's quite easy, really! I went to France and had an artist do some modern painting, and I bought them for £200 each. Then I threw them away and wrote myself receipts for £2,000 each. You don't have to produce the buyer himself, you just book it as cash sale. And sometimes when I was into bigger amounts of money I did it more often.

Then, having been paid in pounds sterling for the cannabis and having sold the cars used for the importation, they exchanged the pounds for French francs. This gave the couple documentation apparently sourcing their income to French art sales, rather than to Britain. We look at money laundering in more detail in Chapter 5.

How common are sideliners?

Sideliners are a problematic category for the researcher, and for drug enforcement agencies. They occupy a logical space within the system of drug distribution, yet by virtue of their legitimate base, resources and channels and the hypothesised infrequency of their involvement, they are particularly hard to detect, contact or research (cf Ruggiero 1990a; 1990b). Yet as Bing Spear, a former Chief Inspector at the Home Office Drugs Branch, observed, the legitimate business traveller with no established connections with the drug market is ideally placed to carry out a drug smuggling run.

> If you are a nice law-abiding citizen, being a nice normal respectable person the chances of you getting pulled coming through Heathrow, Gatwick or Dover, carrying a small quantity, are slim. You can come in with a small amount and if you've got the means of getting rid of it, you can make enough to retire on. (personal communication 1988)

And as a senior intelligence officer concurred:

> I am sure that there are a great many people who are to all intents and purposes licit fronts. . . . I think that there is quite a worrying, silent, blind involvement that doesn't emerge because they are not criminally connected. I mean, of course, they're criminally connected by their activities but they are able to distance themselves from the criminal fraternity.

Research conducted by Waymont and Wright indicates that police drug squad officers estimate that 'legal business people who begin to trade in drugs as a sideline' make up less than 2 per cent of the drug market (Waymont and Wright 1989: section 4). Our own guess is that this is a substantial underestimate, reflecting the greater difficulty of identifying such targets. During our research we were told specific things about a number of medium-sized to large businesses in towns and cities in England, and to repeat those things would definitely be libellous.

Let us turn then to the category of drug trafficker which is estimated by Waymont and Wright's drug squad respondents to make up about half the traffickers that they were dealing with in the late 1980s: the criminal diversifiers.

Chapter 3

Things get nasty
Enter the criminal diversifier

This chapter describes the entry into the drug market of professional criminals from the 1970s onwards. This development has been widely remarked upon by general commentators and by enforcement specialists (Campbell 1990).

> I don't think I'm being over-simplistic here, but probably if you analysed the drug trafficker twenty years ago, he *was* a drug trafficker as opposed to a criminal being diversely engaged. . . . As I said, I've got twenty-odd years' service and my recollection is that there were certain types of people . . . who were into drug trafficking as opposed to *now* when you can clearly see that they are people who are in it because of, one, their criminality; two, their entrepreneurial skills. In other words they see a market and they wish to use that market and also they've become more flexible themselves. They're prepared to move out of extortion and they're prepared to be multi-faceted in their own environments of criminality.
>
> (senior intelligence officer, interview 1989)

Criminological accounts of the roguish entrepreneuriality of small-time crooks and big-time criminals have enjoyed a certain vogue (cf Hobbs 1988; Taylor 1984; Foster 1990).[3] Some of the spirit of their readiness 'to do a deal' in anything is found in the following quote from Frank, a drug dealer turned police informer, telling us that dealing in drugs is no different to dealing in anything else.

> The opportunity – it doesn't matter if it's in time, money, resources, commodities or what it is . . . the phone might ring and it might be saying 'do you know anybody who wants

5 million post cards?' or 'anybody who wants three lorry loads of car parts?' It's a criminal thing going on without drugs.

Frank's case fits the portrait of the kind of 'villain' that Lewis describes as having a familiarity with drug use from their teenage years.

> The involvement of British professional criminals in drug supply may be traced to the 1960s when future 'villains' participated as teenagers in a 'pill' culture that was part of youthful nightlife in the capital. Their familiarisation with amphetamine and cannabis as consumers led eventually to their participation in the developing drugs business.
>
> (Lewis 1989: 42)

Their shift from hedonistic drug consumption into calculating drug trafficking is attributed by some commentators to two principal factors – the increased danger that armed robberies will meet a response from armed police officers, and the recognition that drug trafficking and distribution can yield a very high return. The case of James Hussey and Tommy Wisbey, two members of the gang that carried out the Great Train Robbery in 1963, illustrates this well. As Rose (1988: 8) suggests, their subsequent involvement, over twenty years later, in a large-scale cocaine deal, 'stands as a neat symbol of the changing nature of organised crime' (cf Sweeney 1990: 19).

> Armed robbery . . . has not disappeared. But as the police have shown their willingness to translate intelligence of a robbery into ambushes in which at least five robbers have been shot dead in London alone since February [1988], it has become dangerous and unfashionable. The profits from the drugs trade dwarf the proceeds of all but the very biggest robberies. Such funds . . . can be concealed or laundered far more readily than identifiable banknotes or bullion.
>
> (Rose 1988: 8)

We have already, in the preceding chapter, looked at the link between the participation of established criminals in drug trafficking and the laundering of the proceeds through otherwise legitimate business sideliners.

Sarah and Pete from Metroplace recall the growing involvement of local crime 'gangs' in the drug trade as the market opened up in the north-west. Historically, criminal families had grown up around the docks and canal wharf areas of Metroplace and their business was of a 'traditional' nature. However, as drugs became a more profitable commodity it became ever more tempting to get involved. As Sarah and Pete remember it, such involvement seemed initially to be slow and cautious, 'with some dabbling in the '70s'. However there was no doubt that heavier financial involvement followed in the 1980s. One example given was of robberies carried out abroad with the proceeds then used to buy heroin to increase the profit generated back home. But this was emphatically a business enterprise and 'the gangs didn't like their members to use [the drug], they got elbowed if they did'. Necessary 'street' expertise about quality, weight and the like could easily be hired or, perhaps more likely, pressed into service.

> Any junkie, if they owe money, can be pressured into smuggling or else just to go and test the quality.

In this latter instance, the person would go with members of the firm to represent the principals at the point of exchange and verify that the quality of the drug is as promised. Thus in certain cases apparently small-scale user-dealers may become enmeshed in quite significant transactions and if apprehended, where they are closer to the drugs than the principals, they may end up receiving heavy sentences by default.

Dick and Carla, from north London, confirm that the heroin dealers

> with the most money, don't take it [the drug] themselves . . . they're your villains. They, like, use the proceeds from armed robberies . . . they get into it in a big way and they lay it out on the street in ounces or whatever.

Case study: two 'family firms'

These are two medium-scale organisations, the Bennetts and the Morgans, both with a family history of involvement in traditional crimes such as post office and security van robberies. They were not inter-related (professionally or personally) but, as is common, were described by one police officer as being 'unlikely to step on each other's toes'.

For criminal diversifiers, an essential element of their move into drug distribution is the establishment of contact with an intermediary who provides access to sources of supply. Such facilitators may, however, find their usefulness is short-lived, partly because they are 'outsiders', potentially weak links between the principals involved. This is illustrated in this case, where both families were employing the same intermediary. This was unfortunate for them as this link man subsequently introduced an undercover police officer to them both as a potential multi-kilo buyer of amphetamine sulphate.

The Bennetts are a family described by the police as being 'career criminals'. They epitomise the criminal diversifier of the 1980s, moving from armed robbery to drug distribution as a more profitable and less hazardous outlet for their energies. Bennett senior had recently been released from prison after serving fourteen years for a bank robbery. However, despite the criminal tradition of the family, the lessons of experience are not easily passed on and his son, Malcolm, has been something of a liability, 'shouting his mouth off' about a deal for which he was eventually arrested and convicted. Described by the police as 'a bit of a gobby sod', he

> had recently been elevated from being a snotty burglar kid to the big time. His Dad took him on, meets with good villains and Malcolm couldn't help gobbing off to his former peers. . . . The son is controlled by his father, the son does the negotiating, does the selling [of amphetamine] on the instructions of his father.
>
> (drug squad officer)

Being 'known to the police' in this almost intimate way clearly creates problems for a family firm such as this. They are likely to find that police attention is regularly focused upon them, even at times when they may not actually be involved in any kind of criminal enterprise. In order to retain the necessary room for manoeuvre and the ability to mount a job, a firm has to develop some sophistication in its methods. One example of this is illustrated by the tactics employed to evade police surveillance. The core of this family firm is the father and son but they would also employ ex-robber partners for various jobs, including anti-surveillance work. These hired helps may be assigned to follow a vehicle to check the movements of certain investigating officers or to 'clock' a local police station to note its routine and the regular comings and goings. Communication between members of the observation team would be maintained by mobile telephone whilst 'every villain worth his salt has a "Bearcat" multi-channel radio scanner' for monitoring police radio wavebands (drug squad officer). The fee for a morning's work along these lines might be around £100. As the investigating drug squad officer said, 'the father has the expertise and friends to take out [render useless] police surveillance units and suss out the situation' (cf Lyman 1987: 65).

Other members of the family also played their parts. For example, in the planning stages of one operation the father employed his fourteen-year-old daughter in his anti-surveillance strategy.

> She would go to the police station . . . and at this stage probably just make a mental picture of the vehicles. Near any station you have the policemen who work there who park their cars in the side streets . . . so she makes a mental picture of the regular vehicles. On the day of the meet [to make the deal], she would be sent out of the house very early in the morning because they all know that policemen start dead early in the morning for some reason. She is then equipped with a book and pen [and] goes around looking for any unusual-looking vehicles. She was a shrewd cow, she knew what vehicles to look for. She would then take down the make, the colour and the number. She knows what to look for . . . every police surveillance vehicle is full of McDonald's wrappers in the back. She wouldn't be able to see any radios because they are concealed. She would jot down those numbers [and] include them in the already running card index system . . . from previous criminal enterprises. The father and son would be made aware of these [and] the information passed to the henchmen. This is to forestall the police operation.
>
> (drug squad officer)[4]

Information about the existence, or progress, of any such police operation directed against them may be derived from corrupt, former serving officers who can still pick up a little information or gossip.

> The friends of the defendants were all outside the court . . . straightaway I recognised an ex-detective constable who was thrown out for corruption, in with them! Now where do they get information from? This prat – simple isn't it?

The lifestyle of Bennett senior and family was described by our police respondent in the following terms (cf Hobbs 1988; Taylor 1984)

> [He] draws social security [but is] very affluent, had all the material things in life. . . . The house, you know, they've got a poster from every area of Spain they have been to. The flock wallpaper, the expensive three-piece suite, the nodding donkey bar where you lift its head up and it's got all the drinks inside it. [He's] working class by way of upbringing and education, but purely on finances he is up in the bracket of the middle class. . . . He is the sort of guy who will sit in expensive restaurants with all the gold bangles . . . and he will bring out the biggest wad of notes you have ever seen in your life and buy everyone a drink. I usually call him the 'second-hand car dealer' type of character.

Apart from occasionally smoking cannabis, illegal drug use does not feature greatly in this lifestyle. Drugs are simply a commodity among these 'thorough business men'. Similarly for example, writing about the shooting of Charlie Wilson, one of the Great Train Robbers, Sweeney (1990: 19) made the point that, 'Wilson may perhaps have combined a personal abstinence with a professional interest in drug trafficking'.

The second firm, the Morgans consists of three men. The person who would open preliminary negotiations about a deal is the 'runner' of the firm, David. After leaving school David trained as a builder, eventually became self-employed and, by all accounts, ran a legitimate and successful business. As a juvenile he had one or two brushes with the law for minor offences but otherwise had no criminal record.

By contrast, the senior partner in this firm, Garry, is very well known to the police as 'a bank robber, he has got real pedigree . . . a very, very bad man'. Some years earlier, Garry had been charged with attempted murder after a shooting incident related to a drug deal. But, while he was awaiting trial, his associates threatened the victim who then refused to give evidence. Garry was eventually sentenced to three years' imprisonment for firearms offences.

The third member of the gang is also 'well-known' to the police. Colin is in his mid-to-late thirties and has a long history of involvement in petty and serious crime which has drawn police interest. Beginning with juvenile theft, like 'stealing milk money' and 'doing telephone boxes', he moved into an adult career in armed bank robbery and then, more recently, into a less clearly defined involvement in drug dealing. Another officer in this case said of his arrest that, 'I couldn't believe that we'd got him . . . we used to know him for stealing milk bottles.' Colin is married with two children and has a business as a second-hand car dealer in partnership with Garry, although the business does not seem to have any formal or fixed sales outlet.

Colin's role in the firm was that of trusted holder and deliverer of the drugs, leaving David to set up the deal and Garry to oversee negotiations without either of them having actually to hold the drugs. Such a simple division of labour enhances security against police operations as the most serious point of danger would be if all three participants were to come together with the drugs and with their customers and their cash. However, the routinely security-conscious deal will take place in such a way that the drugs and the money are not actually brought together at the same time in the same place, at all. For the police, 'We have strict rules that the money and the drugs never ever come together' (drug squad officer). Rather, the exchanges take place at different sites with communication enabled by mobile phones.

The story of an undercover officer posing as a buyer to the Bennetts and the Morgans is told in Chapter 6.

Criminal diversifiers in Dublin and Manchester

Eileen, who had moved from Dublin to Manchester, was in a position to provide a picture of criminal diversification and the broader dealing scene in both cities. Indeed, she was quite certain that it was the involvement of the criminal diversifiers in drug distribution in Dublin in the 1980s that was virtually the sole reason for the growth of a serious heroin problem throughout the whole city. About ten years ago, she recalled,

> Dublin, in particular, was flooded with heroin over a period of seven or eight years, mainly through criminal families who previously were not involved in drugs but were mainly into banks and jeweller's shops or whatever and then when they saw the money that was to be made in Dublin they very quickly got in on the scene. Prior to that, the heroin scene in Dublin was a gentle affair, not a lot of real heroin around. . . . [But]

when these families took over, it [heroin] was immediately cut to a low quality, the prices were doubled almost overnight and Dublin became, in a short space of time, what they termed on television, 'the heroin capital of Europe'. Very young people were getting involved and it was a very messy affair.

When Eileen moved to Manchester she was surprised at the scale of the heroin scene there but also remembers being struck by the number of people 'mainly white – in a way a bit similar to Dublin – of a criminal background who got in on the drugs thing. . . . But the main dealers who were doing ounces and above didn't seem to be users themselves'. The background of the new heroin traffickers was that of the established criminal.

People who are into robbing banks or into armed robberies per se and over the years the police have been getting pretty good at catching these people and more police are being armed, [so] to be on the street with a gun, out to get money, is walking on very narrow [sic] ice at the moment. 'Cause if you were caught you were going down for it and it's a big sentence and then suddenly heroin comes along and it's a very easy way of making quick money. And all you need is a contact and if you've got the money behind you, well then you start like, you're in business, it's not something that you have to learn or that there's a lot to learn about. Like you're in business once you've got a contact and if you've got money and if you've got the bottle to do it, then why not? And, I'm sure, at the time, the Serious Crime Squad probably had a sigh of relief, as I know they did in Dublin, when the raids on banks went down or people being held up for money or jewellery or whatever, when that dropped – in particular in Dublin – they, the criminals, were given a lot of rope to get in on the drugs scene – and perhaps too much and that was why it got so serious. And, I think, perhaps not on the same scale, it happened here, maybe serious crime dropped in terms of arms, guns and that.

These established, criminal elements are directly involved in importation as well as local sale.

I mean I came in contact with some people recently who are involved in, we'll say, other forms of crime, other than drugs, and they have just recently got involved in drugs and their shipments are coming from Spain and they are on a regular basis, bringing in, a few kilos a week of heroin and also Spanish amphetamine . . . they've been bringing in these two substances . . . successfully now for about six months via couriers. They're not shipping it in massive bulk, but they're sending couriers regularly every week. And that's well organised, it'll probably be in the form of families going. But I suppose, again, sooner or later, that's going to be cottoned on to.

Typically, according to Eileen, the 'contact' easing entry into the drug distribution business would be a local person, with a long history of drug dealing, who may or may not be a user themselves but if they are will not be using to the extent that they are 'strung out'. It is likely that they will be 'making a lot of money' but will be doing so sufficiently discreetly to have had little, if any, trouble with the law (or at least will not have been in prison). They may previously have 'been looked down on' by local villains but 'if people around them are going up for big sentences 'cause they're holding up security vans or whatever', then dealing can suddenly seem quite attractive. Then, as the business builds and the money flows, 'what tends to happen is that the local contact is eventually got offside and then they take over themselves as soon as they know the ins and outs'.

Violence and firearms

The pressures which led criminals familiar with intimidation and violence to move into the drug market, from the 1970s onwards, have transformed the 'climate' of drug trafficking. It is not purely nostalgic to observe that drug dealing in the 'good old days' of the 1960s occurred in circumstances of personal safety. This has to some extent now changed, though the extent of change varies from one part of Britain to another.

In London, the new professionalism of the 1980s is typified by a firm originally from the north-west. The nucleus of this firm all had criminal backgrounds in vice and gambling. They had been coming down to London looking for contacts and outlets.

In a very short time, they are here, they are slotted into the community, they make various contacts, they obtain various vehicles . . . [and] various addresses and safe addresses.

(drug squad officer)

The addresses were empty properties, used to supply to other dealers and to some user-dealers. Having a base in London the firm was also observed spreading into other cities, establishing a reputation as they went along for being highly organised and businesslike. For example, they were involved in a shooting over a rip-off.

> This firm is so well organised that when somebody ripped them off and left the city they worked from [and] came down under an assumed identity and set up his own business front, they found out where he was and shot him dead.
>
> (drug squad officer)

And their attitude to business is summed up as, 'If you are good for business then you are good for business'.

In Manchester, Eileen relates that

> [The dealers' tools now are] a car-phone and, in quite a lot of cases, a gun. Especially when they are out on the estates and they are carrying a large amount of heroin. There is a never-ending feud coming over from North Manchester, where there was a spate of shootings a few months ago where there was nearly a shooting every night of the week for something like a month. Somebody would come over and shoot somebody over here and it seemed to be more people were being shot over here than [another district]. And that was all to do with dealing and women.
>
> Q. So one of the things that's changed in your time in Manchester is the level of violence then?
>
> Yes, definitely. There are more and more stories of incidents where doors have been kicked in and a small army's steamed in. I actually witnessed one of them and that was very, very nasty, to be stood in a room in front of a gang of people with baseball bats and swords and I think one of them also had a gun. And that's happening very readily. It's not a nice scene to be involved in.

Even if much of this is indeed just the stuff of local 'stories', it none the less reflects a strong perception of the violent and rough nature of the dealing scene today – a perception which has real consequences as people involved come to expect violence or employ it themselves on the expectation that otherwise others will direct it toward them. It seems probable that excitable British media coverage of greater degrees of violence by drug traffickers and law enforcement agents in the United States has a similar effect. We are moving into a time when it is easy to make negative predictions come true.

CONCLUDING OBSERVATIONS

It is worth observing that frequently in discussing diversifiers, and their links to sideliners, the importance of *family* ties was emphasised by many of our respondents. A sizeable distribution operation might extend across a city, across the country or involve links with others in a different country, but in many cases the strength and security of these enterprises relies on keeping power and control close to the domestic hearth. As one London police officer described it

> So you'd have groups of people who'd established contacts in places and operate on a very large scale [but] their distribution network is purely domestic usually. You know, friends of the family and relatives of them and so on and so forth who are allowed to know the family's business.

The characterisation of a firm as a 'family concern' does not mean that activity is confined to close blood relatives, rather it is a certain ethos and set of binding values that are being referred to. With the hardening of markets, the security of the real or adopted family is a safe haven for some people. As the 1980s progressed, however, other people took a different, more individualistic path – trusting no one.

Chapter 4

Contested streets
Retailing into the 1990s

Throughout this study, we emphasise the fragmentary and fluid nature of drug markets. Stable drug trafficking organisations, as described in the preceding chapter, are often one- or two-person affairs, and rarely bigger than five or six, regardless of the amount of drugs they trade. The occasional big seizures by the enforcement agencies do not mean big organisations.

In this chapter, we look further down market, to the more temporary and sometimes unstable sorts of organisations that arose at the retail level of the market during the 1980s. We also examine how some of these recently formed enterprises move up market, trafficking in larger amounts whilst not changing their basic structure very much. Others, of course, get apprehended by drug enforcement agencies, leaving a gap in the market that is usually refilled within a few months (Reuter *et al*. 1990).

The first type of retailer that we describe, the opportunistic irregulars, may best be thought of as younger, less experienced and more erratic versions of the established criminals described in Chapter 3: they participate in a wide variety of petty crimes, regarding drugs as one of many commodities. They can be thought of as being 'self-employed', albeit in primarily illegal markets.

The second type of organisation, the retail specialists, can be regarded as illegal enterprises paralleling legitimate firms in which labour is hired by the hour, day or week, or on a profits-sharing basis. It is this latter type that characterises retail-level trafficking in many North American cities, and increasingly announced itself in Britain throughout the 1980s.

Both types of operations present a relatively publicly visible spectacle, sometimes threatening the public's sense of tranquillity and safety, and have become the target of intense police pressure.

As we shall describe in Part II of this book, drug policies and policing strategies increasingly target the point of retail purchase, aiming to reduce the availability of drugs at the retail end of the market, or to increase the time which customers must spend in searching out sellers of drugs. If purchasers can be put to more trouble, the idea is, then maybe they will think twice about their purchase, and hence have nothing to consume ('inconvenience policing'). Another, related way of attending to the point of sale is to harry the customer, for example by making arrests of those who have purchased drugs for personal use. This is sometimes presented as a form of 'demand reduction'. The renewed attention being given to policing the drug trade at retail level is partly a fall-back strategy, resulting from disappointment over the limited success of strategies targeting 'the big trafficking organisations' (a disappointment which, for us, necessarily follows from the absence of this type). The success or otherwise of this control emphasis depends upon the extent to which the dealers have the flexibility to evolve their modus operandi and stay ahead of the game.

OPPORTUNISTIC IRREGULARS: JUMP-UP MERCHANTS

Irregulars are individuals or groups, small or large, who respond to short-term market opportunities as these arise. They eschew long-term planning, involving themselves in the multi-commodity trading to be found in 'street culture', the networking of those on the club scene of any city, or the quiet negotiations conducted in the corners of countless bars (Henry 1978; Hobbs 1988). They may or may not consume drugs, and in any case such consumption is not their over-riding concern. Rather, money, excitement and recognition in the street culture and local social networks are the goals. Our street entrepreneurs and hustlers in this category are relatives of what Hobbs calls 'the jump-up merchant'.

> The term 'jump-up' itself comes from the literal description of a person who follows delivery vans and lorries until the driver stops to make a delivery, and at an opportune moment our stalking hero 'jumps up' and grabs whatever he can.
>
> (Hobbs 1988: 158)

Operating within the shady area of activity that Henry (1978) has called 'borderline crime', the irregular, like the jump-up merchant, 'does not differentiate between legal and illegal opportunities and with few exceptions will judge an opportunity according to potential profit and loss' (Hobbs 1988: 155).

If the enterprise brings with it additional profit calculable not just in terms of cash but also in terms of social status and a bit of a laugh, then so much the better. A respondent interviewed in prison describes an area of London that he knows well and the attractions of taking up an 'irregular' opportunity.

> You see a lot of the people that make money on the streets . . . [in this area] they're either barrow people [from the street markets], second-hand car salesmen, this sort of thing. They like a flutter, a game of cards. Now the people they're playing cards with, [in] all-night sessions and drinking with in the clubs or pubs that they use, are up-and-coming people that are earning money off drugs or off the street itself, they're street-wise people, and to mingle one lot of money with another lot of money is no problem. They're either washing money, or they're using bookies or they get in a bit of debt or somebody says, 'listen, I'm going to Amsterdam', then they say, 'where're you getting that money from?' – 'Oh, well we've just made a nice trip, scoring' – 'Well, how much have you got there?' – 'Well, we made twenty grand you know, and we had a couple of weeks out there as well and blew a bit of bread'.

The availability of many legal and semi-legal businesses in the commercial infrastructure of the locality provides easy channels for laundering sudden windfalls of income.

The review of 'the social organisation of drug dealing among urban gangs' by Fagan (1989: 633–67) offers examples of gangs fitting here. For example, Feldman et al. (1985) describe 'entrepreneurial gangs'. These were identified in a study of Latino gangs in San Francisco and 'consisted of youths who were concerned with attaining social status by means of money and the things money can buy'.

During the late 1980s, one prominent image of drug traffickers presented by the mass media was the black male in the form of the 'yardie', represented as erratic and violence prone in their actions to the point of dangerousness (Sweeney 1989: 27–30). Clearly, this is an image of trafficking in which racist stereotyping is prominent (File on Four 1990). Within Britain, trafficking was acknowledged as a predominantly white business up until the 1980s, but from the middle of the decade onwards race emerged as a recurrent motif in the debate on trafficking. Eileen, an informed observer of the Manchester scene, herself white, gives her perspective on the changes that have taken place.

As we know now, the whole scene changed fairly quickly where it became centralised in central Manchester, in particular in Moss Side where I noticed that more and more people that I knew as users, the source that they were getting their heroin from was from black dealers on the street in Moss Side and everybody very, very quickly, though not willingly, fell into the pattern of 'if you want heroin, then you go to the Moss and in particular you go to the precinct' where at any one time there would be between one and perhaps forty black dealers and that is without any exaggeration.

The shift from domination of the market by white criminal families (as described in Chapter 3) and white 'irregulars' to a market also involving black groups was partly attributed to

The way in which they [black dealers] made heroin available to the point where they were very blatantly and openly selling heroin in the shopping centre, on the streets, whereas . . . white dealers would probably do it from a house or a pub or have what they call runners, running around the district doing bits and pieces for them. And, if they decide to go anywhere or even go away, well that source has dried up or if there's a drought that source is gone and people have to go elsewhere to find drugs. [Whereas] if you walk into Moss Side centre and drug dealers are queuing up to sell you drugs. Well, there's one of the attractions. It's there all the time.

Another white observer attributes the increase in involvement of black people in dealing as resulting from the denial of legitimate opportunities.

It's a fast way to make money. I mean it's a community that has been suppressed, oppressed, for a long time and has suddenly found a way to be above the white man in a lot of respects. Especially in the areas that they live in, most people don't have cars or telephones or whatever or expensive clothes, but now you go round Moss Side and you look at the black people and they are very well dressed and they're driving very nice cars and they're not going to let these material things go. They haven't had them for a long time and now they've got them and they're going to keep them. And I would imagine what's most enjoyable about that is that the people who are funding their luxuries are white people and historically it's been the white people who've deprived them of many luxuries – so it must be a right buzz for them to be in that position.

Whether or not this accurately reflects the motivational accounts that would be given by black traffickers in this locale is a matter which cannot be pronounced upon here. Perhaps more work should be done, but there is little *a priori* reason to attribute to black traffickers a range of motivations different from those of whites. It might perhaps be the case that racism in the drug market has for many years kept it a primarily white preserve – in which case one would have to explain why such exclusionary processes have only recently been overcome. One hypothesis that was offered to us was that the Manchester police may have reasoned that the drug trade was unstoppable, and that since it was bound to happen somewhere, it might as well happen in black areas – leading to a tacit policy of differential enforcement. Of course, such suggestions are denied by the city police, who also point out that when they *do* carry out operations in black areas, some people allege racism. (We return to questions of policing local drug markets in Chapter 7.)

Interestingly, rivalry between groups from different areas was mentioned but generally as occurring *within* the different ethnic communities rather than between them.

> They [the white and black gangs] tend to keep away from each other. It's that sort of respect, you know, 'you don't bother us, we don't bother you'. And that's the way it seems to work unless that's infringed upon and if somebody does cross that line, *then* something happens.
>
> (Eileen)

The implication is that both white and black irregulars accept skin colour as a useful way of delineating spheres of influence. This is in contrast to other aspects of the city's culture, for example many of its leading music clubs, where 'Acid House' and its derivatives in the 1980s are said to have had a clearly multi-racial character. The politics of race then seem to be represented in different ways in different sites.

Generally speaking, those we have described as irregulars, whether white or black, tend to be attracted by the short-term deal and take more of a gamble on the resulting pay-off. They are primarily male. Our next category of trafficker, by contrast, 'retail specialists' think organisationally and in the medium to long term. Although still a minority, women do occupy roles within the latter type of enterprise. There are signs that both these ways of operating expanded in Britain during the 1980s.

RETAIL SPECIALISTS

Retail specialists tend to be fairly stable, hierarchical, commercially organised operations. They will have a managerial structure of some kind (in North American studies referred to as being headed by a 'crew boss') and 'employees' will perform a range of specialised tasks, for example, to protect the merchandise, delivering small deals, collecting payment, ensuring security by keeping lookout, seeking to mislead or divert investigative authorities and competition and so on (cf Preble and Casey 1969; Johnson *et al.* 1985; Williams 1989). In other words they mirror many of the things that a competitive legitimate commercial enterprise might do.

In the past this kind of structure has been more evident in the major urban centres of North America (cf Moore 1977) than in Britain. However, in the mid-1980s, Pearson (1987: 127–8) found evidence of smaller scale but similar divisions of labour in Manchester and in Liverpool. One of our own respondents also described the use of lookouts and diversionary tactics on Merseyside:

> They'll have their joeys [helpers] all over the place [and] one or two people who are your protectors . . . if you get bust on the street, they'll do their best to cause a commotion or fight to give you a chance to drop it on the street or do a runner.
>
> (Jane)[5]

This kind of arrangement is now becoming more common in Britain. A typical arrangement was described by a senior officer with a brief to monitor the market in crack.

> [There will be] a mastermind, with runners, many of them young, spotters, [with] the stash somewhere else, very little on the person. . . . The 'washing up' [converting cocaine into

rocks of crack] takes place in an empty flat across the road
and this place is changed quite frequently. Then it's taken to
a particular stash point holding, say, ten rocks, where a person
goes to pick them up for sale.

Employees in such outfits may or may not be drug users themselves
– the important organisational imperative is that they are not
'stoned' whilst working as this would impair efficiency. This is
well described in research on organisations of adolescent crack
sellers in Detroit that prohibited drug use among their members
(Cooper 1987). As Fagan summarises

> Leaders in these groups were wary of both threats to efficiency
> and security if street-level sellers were high and the potential
> for corruption of their business goals if one of their members
> became a consumer of their goods. The gangs were organised
> around income, and they saw drug use as detracting from the
> selling skills and productivity of the members.
>
> (Fagan 1989: 636–7)

A similar prohibition was found to apply in a different study of
street-level adolescent drug runners in heroin dealing organisations
(Mieczkowski 1986). Recreational use of marijuana and cocaine
was permissible in social situations removed from the dealing
scene; however, penalties of either a violent or economic nature
were imposed by 'crew bosses' if the rules were broken.

In the retail specialist organisations that we describe below, the
pattern of usage by the dealers themselves was variable. In one
organisation all three including the head, Ian, were using heroin
and crack. However, the people who worked with them were
usually, but not necessarily, users. In two other organisations,
the managers – Billy and Jeff – were not and apparently never
had been users themselves. Both of the other two team members
working with Jeff were heroin users. Of Billy's team, Mike is said to
'have liked his bit of coke', but Francis and John were not thought
to be users, apparently preferring to consume in other conspicuous
ways: 'They're just car and jewellery crazy' (Jane).

Successful retail organisations often reproduce the organisational
division of labour to be found in legitimate sales-oriented businesses. The Welch organisation, tried in 1988 for the smuggling
and dealing of cocaine and cannabis, provides an example. Welch
planned and led the gang, while his girlfriend was described by the

judge as 'the gang's accountant', who 'became a very competent manager of the day-to-day affairs of this organisation'. A third defendant, Dennis Wheeler, whose legal profession was as a sales manager, was described in court as 'an international cannabis merchant responsible for financing, organising and shipping the cargo'. Six others played lesser roles in the organisation as carriers, labourers and so on (Horsnell 1988: 3).

Other features which can be likened to a legitimate business model of operations can be identified in the operation of retail specialists. One of these is to discipline the buyers into knowing when the dealer's 'office hours' are. Just as shops and businesses will trade only during set hours, dealers who want to establish a reasonable degree of control over their clientele will work to established patterns. These 'office hours' are particularly important for those dealing from a fixed or static location, like a house or flat, because the alternative would be the prospect of being continually 'on call' to buyers, potentially a very disruptive existence.

For example, Ian, Oliver and Scott were a three-man team, all in their mid-to-late twenties who were supplying heroin on a London council estate. Ian and Oliver were unemployed, Scott was working as a truck operator. All of them have very long criminal records for a range of petty and serious offences including the possession and supply of controlled drugs. They worked in a straightforward vertical hierarchy with Ian in charge, Oliver the deputy leader and Scott as the junior. This team operated from the flat of Ian's parents, who knew what was going on but were not otherwise involved, apart from, as one police officer put it, 'just happening to get two hundred quid a night' (for the use of the flat). All three would turn up separately at about 6.00 p.m. by which time a queue of buyers was beginning to form underneath a first-floor window. Scott, as 'the donkey' in this team, would come down and take money from the buyers, go back into the house and the paid-for quantity of heroin would be dropped in a bag from the first-floor window. They would sell to between twenty and twenty-five people every evening and worked up to about 10.00 p.m. Two slight variations on this basic method were observed by the police. Oliver, described as 'a bit shrewder' (than Scott), would take people into an alleyway round the corner when supplying directly. On other occasions, Ian could be observed in the entrance to the flat, where he would 'unwind the cellophane and stand there and dish it out'.

People knew when they were open and [when] they close. People knew it was a heroin shop, they knew the hours, [if you came late] you couldn't get it.

(drug squad officer)

This feature of openness of this static dealing organisation is confirmed by the remark that 'Ian was the worst kept secret around, everyone knew he was dealing, everyone told us he was dealing . . . when we arrested [them], there was people clapping'. When the case came to trial, all three pleaded guilty to conspiracy to supply heroin. Ian received a sentence of six years, Scott got five years, and Oliver five years (including sentence for possessing a shotgun and the invocation of a previous suspended sentence).

Houses and streets

A different sort of retailing operation, found in a north-western city, is described by another informant. Here Billy is the manager. Two of the 'intermediaries' (Mike and Francis) are related to Billy (nephews). The third intermediary, John, is Billy's friend. The three intermediaries control a greater number of street dealers. At the time of our interview with Jane (who previously worked with them) they had been working within this structure for about five years.

Billy, though clearly known as the manager or head of the organisation, had distanced himself by one step from the actual supplying. This reflects police opinion that 'good dealers don't handle the stuff themselves'. Billy would travel to buy the stuff from London but the street and house dealers would be supplied by the three intermediaries: 'you'd see them dropping and picking money up and things, being joeys'. It was they who would 'drop off' supplies to the houses and street dealers. Billy's 'patch' focused upon

one cul-de-sac on an estate and he had about five houses working for him and about eight lads out on the street working for him. That's just one dealer so you're talking about one leader having anything from ten to fifteen people working for him . . . they were selling heroin and freebase cocaine.

(Jane)

The house dealers worked from their own residences and buyers came to the house to purchase drugs. The workers were supplied on a 'supply and demand system [where] when [one] load's gone out you re-stock' (drug agency worker).

> The people on the estate would get a quarter of an ounce a day to sell and if it went before the day was out they could have another one, so that was like five quarters on the estate. Maybe some people would get rid of half an ounce of heroin a day, but . . . we sold a lot more coke, [it's in] much larger quantities.
>
> (Jane)

Street dealers work to their own patch, demarcated by street corners, cafés and street furniture such as lamp posts. Competition for customers can be intense and is manifested in two ways:

> If you're walking up the street anything from five to ten people will approach you . . . showing it to you in bags, mainly heroin and coke. They get to know your own punters and they're called soldiers when they're out on the street and if another soldier approaches your punter there's absolute murder. You have like your own set of punters. But the sellers will always try to get other buyers, obviously the more they sell the better the turnover for them.
>
> (Jane)

The competition for particular spaces and customers is complemented by a form of advertising. In this case it is the house dealers who are competing for custom.

> There's five in that close and they'll sit on the wall outside the house and say 'oh come over here my bag is bigger than his' or 'they've got shit gear, I've got clean gear', that sort of bartering going on.
>
> (Jane)

The workers or soldiers were recruited through different sources, some being users themselves, others were people who knew Billy and were looking for some work. 'We used to call them "breadheads", you know people who used to want to make money but don't mind taking high risks at making it'. The soldiers were both white and black and about equal numbers were male and female.

Billy's operation follows the classic small business entrepreneurship model.

Billy had started with a few grams and just gone up and up, the more money he's had the larger quantities he's bought in and the more quantity you have the more power it gives them.

(Jane)

This retail specialist operation also demonstrates aspects of opportunism and an eye for the market. From an interest in and attendance at horse racing meetings, Billy developed his operation, supplying drugs on a race course.

Distribution by delivery

Another retail level organisation, this time providing mobile sales outlets, consists of Jeff as the head and Sharon and Barry as the two workers. All three lived in south-east London, were in their mid-twenties and unemployed. Jeff and Barry had never had any employment, while Sharon had previously worked in a variety of routine factory jobs. Sharon had a long criminal record of mainly petty offences (theft/shoplifting) as well as drug possession offences. Barry had previous juvenile (taking and driving away automobiles) and burglary offences. Jeff had previous convictions for possessing an offensive weapon and for obstructing a drug search.

In court, Barry said that he had been using heroin since the age of seventeen or eighteen, consuming between a half and three-quarters of a gram a day. Sharon was also a long-term heroin user, who had been injecting, unlike Barry, who used only by 'chasing the dragon'. The two workers received money and heroin as payment in kind from Jeff. Their method of working entailed receiving calls on a pager displaying telephone numbers which buyers could be phoned back on. Pagers could also be used to transmit other urgent messages of course and in one instance Jeff received a warning on his pager telling him to 'back off, the drug squad are after you'! Although there were around 5,000 messages logged on the pager in a period of about ten weeks, this organisation is thought to have only about eighty customers as regular buyers. Most of the buyers bought a quarter or half a gram, but they also sold to other suppliers.

Sharon would call the buyers back and arrange the quantity to be bought and a place for the exchange. She recorded deliveries according to time and place on a note pad. So, for instance, at

11.30 a.m. there would be a list with a first name, a meeting place indicated by initials (for example, BS meant bus stop, P a local park, etc.) and a quantity. She would then weigh out and bag up the heroin and Jeff and Barry would go out to make the deliveries. They had usual hours when they would be making their rounds.

> They normally have times they would supply, it used to be 11 o'clock, 2 o'clock, 6 o'clock and 10 o'clock at night. So around an hour before they were due to go out and supply the calls would start coming in.
>
> (drug squad officer)

Jeff aimed to establish a reputation of providing value for money.

> His measurements were good, good value for money. 250 mg is a lot of weight, the other people are selling 100 mg in [another] road for £20, and he was selling it 250 mg for £25, so he had a lot of business, hence made a lot of money very quickly.

In this case, the eventual removal by the police of such an active entrepreneur had an effect on the streets, though not what might be expected.

> We've not really found anybody who's taken Jeff's place. What we have found is that there are a lot more street dealers coming onto the street, so nobody's operating in the bigger circles like Jeff [used to] at the present time. We've got a mushroom effect and the [main dealing] road has now become very busy again, it's always been busy, [now it's] busier.

This illustrates the perennial problem in policing retail markets – the so-called 'displacement effect'. The removal of Jeff resulted in a quietening of activity for a while, during which users had to look elsewhere for their supplies. This period of inactivity in the road was followed by the 'replacement effect' – the entry into the market of many smaller independent operators.

Yuppie retailing

At the time of interview, Greg was on bail pending an appearance at the Crown Court for his involvement in cocaine dealing. He has lived all his life in the Home Counties and comes from a prosperous middle-class family. He had a poor record of attendance at school and left without any qualifications. At the time that Greg became a school refuser he started hanging around a local recording studio where he did occasional casual work. Through his contact with the owner of the studio he began to purchase small quantities of cannabis and amphetamine and started to deal in these to various friends. He would deal in cannabis in amounts up to one ounce and in amphetamine in up to one gramme.

The studio owner, Maxwell, himself a dealer in sizeable quantities, purchased his supply through contacts in the 'music industry'. Maxwell has always been involved in a little dealing but his studio business was legitimate. In this respect, in terms of his early involvement in dealing and his targeting of customers through his studio, he can be seen as an example of what we call a 'sideliner' (Chapter 2). However, his involvement soon developed far beyond being a dabbling sideline and matured into a highly profitable business, dwarfing other interests. After coming into an unexpected windfall of money, Maxwell decided to move into the cocaine market, obtaining his supplies direct from a Peruvian importer. In his estimation this would be a safe commodity to deal in since the targeted client group would be the everyday users of his recording studio.

Greg's involvement in cocaine dealing came about as an extension of his earlier trade in amphetamine and cannabis – taking half ounces of cocaine on credit from Maxwell and selling one gramme deals to friends and acquaintances. He made his own profit by cutting the coke with cornflour (which does not alter the appearance of the powder). The cocaine supplied to Greg was at least 75 per cent pure and so a one-third cut still gave him a product of about 50 per cent purity. As is usual with the sale of smaller quantities of a product he also added a further price 'mark-up'. With the cut in purity and the price mark-up, Greg could make enough money to pay off Maxwell and make a personal financial profit, and in addition retain enough cocaine for his personal use.

As the cocaine business grew for both of them, Maxwell became more anxious to avoid attracting attention so he withdrew a little, relying more on Greg, who was supplied with larger quantities on credit. At this time they also moved into supplying slightly larger quantities to other dealers and in these transactions Greg was paid an extra commission in lieu of taking a cut out of the cocaine.

The business then expanded to London where Maxwell had many contacts in the music industry. Here the operational procedure changed in a significant way. Now Greg had direct access to Paul, the 'runner' for Mr Smith, the importer from whom Maxwell obtained his bulk supplies. Greg was equipped with a portable phone and based himself on the streets in a business area on the south bank of the Thames. He received calls from customers who placed orders for varying quantities (usually between half an ounce and two ounces) and then, when he had collected sufficient orders, he placed a bulk order (say between two and six ounces of cocaine) with Paul. The order was placed by phone but delivery was by hand. Paul would pick up Greg in his car and hand over the coke which Greg then cut and packaged as Paul drove them around. Greg was then dropped off to call his customers and arrange to meet them for delivery and payment. From the accumulated monies Greg then paid off Paul. Greg worked his patch from 2.00 p.m. to 6.00 p.m. for three or four days a week.

For really large sales, say between eight and sixteen ounces, a different procedure was adopted. Maxwell would supply the money to Greg to make the bulk purchase from Paul. The cocaine would then be supplied more-or-less uncut and Greg and Maxwell would cut it with some inert substance before selling it, then split the profit.

Their modus operandi was considered secure since they had started with customers they knew and were consistent in dealing only with existing customers; if they took on a new customer, this had to be someone who was introduced by a trusted, existing customer. They would not entertain 'cold sales'. In addition, since Greg was only in actual possession of the cocaine for a short period of time this was considered another safeguard. As things turned out however, it was precisely this faith in the security of introductions from regular customers that led to their encounter with a new customer supposedly in search of a supplier for his own client group. This 'dealer' turned out to be an undercover drug squad officer.

Case study: a novice retailer learns quickly

Ari is a middle-class man in his thirties, securely established in his father's business of managing rented property, who saw in the growing local drug scene a means of making extra money. From north London contacts, Ari obtained a couple of ounces of heroin but, unsure of the appropriate marketing practices and unclear about how to identify local customers outside of his tenant group, his initial strategy was flawed with two basic and naive errors.

1 Firstly, he did not cut his material (which was 75 per cent pure in the form he obtained from his supplier) to the normal strength available locally (about 35 per cent purity); and he did not align his price with current market prices. In other words he was selling heroin that was too strong and too cheap. He had calculated his profit as coming solely from a straight mark-up and had ignored the profit to be made from cutting the drug.
2 Secondly, since he did not have access to the majority of potential clients, he also supplied to a couple of his tenants on credit with the idea that they would cut the heroin, sell it onto others and then pay him.

As a result of the first error there followed a number of predictable overdoses suffered by long-term injectors which led in turn to a general move toward smoking this 'new' heroin. Ari gained a reputation for supplying good material at a low price and effectively squeezed other local dealers out of the picture. From the second error, however, he learned that if he was to organise his distribution system successfully to reach all potential customers in the local heroin market, he would need to pick more reliable intermediaries and exert more effective control over them. His first dealers, recruited from among his tenants, had themselves used most of the heroin he had supplied on credit and had then cut the remainder heavily in order to make sufficient profit to repay Ari.

Ari realised that he needed a more professional organisation. He recruited three or four (it varied over time) heroin dealers who knew the local scene, were used to dealing in reasonable sized quantities and who would fill this role on a long-term basis. These were to be his exclusive distributors in the town. Ari would supply them with heroin on a payment-on-sale basis which the dealers would then cut to provide their profit and then sell in one-fifth gramme amounts on a cash basis. Ari's profit came from buying in bulk and selling in smaller lots at a premium price. Now he was working with 'employees' who were used to dealing, unlike his earlier tenant dealers who were basically chaotic users, and stability was achieved. Further, once he had purchased and sold his original consignment of heroin the operation could become self-financing with no cash-flow problems. This was important because Ari's supplier would work only on a cash basis.

Having organised his sales representatives, Ari now brought in members of his family to act as senior management. He recruited his younger brother Jack, who was dissatisfied with the traditional family business, and also his cousin Leo who lived in a nearby town and ran a nightclub. Jack and Leo were to act as managers, minders and contacts with the London suppliers. Leo's nightclub was in a town with a larger population of heroin users and this group was supplied by an already existing network of dealers. Shrewdly, Ari and partners decided they would not seek to compete with the existing petty dealers but, instead, would set up a system of bulk sales to them. So, using Leo's nightclub as a contact and sales point they started to sell lots of 100 grammes to established dealers on a cash-up-front basis. When in full operation – which lasted about two years – the organisation was moving up to one kilo of heroin per week through the two sites.

During these two years, various other younger family members were attracted by the profits involved and joined the operation in minor roles. The senior management of the operation always felt secure because they were buying only from within a close-knit community where police surveillance would be limited. And once they had purchased their supply they never had it in their possession for very long because it was passed to their sales force as soon as possible.

However, Ari and co had a high profile in the community and their identities were well known among local users. Further, they liked high-status consumption. Unlike their parents, Ari's generation did not re-invest their profits in business diversification, but instead they spent it on fast cars, speed boats, portaphones and the club scene. The sales force succumbed to temptation and were using heroin heavily since they had easy access to it at a cheap price. It can be surmised that as a consequence their behaviour breached security and the attention paid to precautions suffered. Interestingly, the senior managers never took to heroin use but Ari and Leo developed cocaine habits using in the order of three to five grammes a day. However, they never diversified their own sales operations into cocaine because they could not purchase it from their contacts or, perhaps, because they did not see it as a drug that they could move through their existing network to their regular heroin-using customers.

Police broke the organisation through a long-term undercover surveillance operation. Surveillance videos of the houses of the sales force and of their clients played a part in the prosecution as did plea bargaining by other minor participants in the organisation who were arrested by the police but never charged. Ari's organisation was something of an anomaly in this area. The dealing scene had ticked over with some consistency before their arrival and it would do so again after, but it seems likely that the legacy of a more business-like approach would linger.

CONCLUSION

In this first part of the book, we have offered some perspectives on the variety of and changes in drug trafficking in Britain over the past three decades. We have tried to draw some rough sketches in broadly social and cultural terms. In describing trafficking, we suggest that what is important is the social background, opportunities, resources, cultures and ways of working of individuals and small groups, who weave in and out of the trade, going up market sometimes, changing how they operate another time, and going back down market or ceasing to trade as circumstances change. Interactions between traffickers and enforcement agencies are one of the principal stimuli to change (cf Dorn and South 1990; George and Fraser 1989; Reuter *et al.* 1988). Drug markets are *messy*.

But there is of course another way of describing drug trafficking, one which corresponds to the popular image. From that perspective, markets are described in terms of a series of hierarchical distribution levels, defined by weights of drugs traded (Wagstaff and Maynard 1988: 53, drawing upon Lewis *et al.* 1985). People are simply kilo dealers, ounce dealers, etc. In its most extreme version, this 'triangular' model of the market is topped by a few groups ('the cartels') or even one group (monopoly). Interactions between traffickers and enforcement agencies may make a slight change to the volumes of drugs traded, but do not have much effect on the social forms that trafficking takes. Drug markets are *simple*. Such a notion appeals because it is simple, easy to grasp, has great entertainment value, is consonant with certain economic theories about markets in general, is likely to generate funding for enforcement agencies – and seems to fit into or mirror the hierarchical organisation of enforcement agencies.

In Britain, where during the 1980s policing was developing into three organisational levels (national/regional, city/county, and local – see ACPO 1985: partially reproduced in the Appendix of this book), it has been found convenient to conceive of trafficking as being similarly organised. (The following three chapters describe some operations at each level of enforcement.) However, the notion that the social organisation of drug markets mirrors the organisation of enforcement can be regarded as no more than a convenient fiction. Later in the study, we suggest that the credibility of this particular fiction is slipping away.

Part II

Enforcement strategies

Chapter 5

Policing from the top down
From US theory to UK practice

Part II of this book describes drug enforcement strategies as operationalised at the upper, middle and local levels of police organisation in Britain. This chapter notes the appeal of a strategy of going for the 'big traffickers' and discusses the way in which this has evolved into a new focus on money laundering. Chapters 6 and 7 will examine policing strategies at the presumed middle and lower levels of the market. We have not made any special study of Her Majesty's Customs and Excise, who are primarily responsible for interdiction at national frontiers, but Chapter 9 looks at drugs intelligence which is one of the areas where cooperation between Customs and police is increasing.

GOING FOR MR BIG

The US example

A major goal of drug enforcement is to climb to the top of 'the pyramid' and arrest the major dealers and organisers who are believed to control the drug trade. In this Mr Big strategy, the 'principal operational objective is to reach high levels of the drug distribution system . . . using wiretaps, informants and undercover activities' (Moore and Kleiman 1989: 6). It is the stated priority of the US Drug Enforcement Administration (henceforth DEA) and during the 1970s and 1980s became accepted world-wide.

> DEA's goal is to reduce the availability of illicit narcotics and dangerous drugs in the domestic marketplace, and to disrupt the drug traffic through the arrest and prosecution of major violators and the removal of their assets.
>
> (Lawn 1985: 31)

But while the idea of Mr Big may be familiar, in practice the questions 'how big is big?' and who qualifies for inclusion in this category have proved problematic. In 1969 the US Bureau of Narcotics and Dangerous Drugs (BNDD), one of the forerunners of the DEA, adopted the 'systems approach' which required all of its regional offices to produce reports and organisational charts on activity in their regions. From this the BNDD constructed major and secondary classification systems for trafficking organisations.

A report by the Comptroller General noted major shortcomings with the BNDD's systems approach: the criteria for identifying major traffickers were not clearly defined and instructions to the regions did not specify criteria. 'The only criterion for measuring the importance of a trafficker was whether immobilization of the trafficker "would make a significant impact on the availability of illicit drugs in the United States"' (US Comptroller General 1976: 10). Not surprisingly, given the tendency for officers to wish to demonstrate some degree of success in their work, subsequent inspection established that this approach leads to some individuals being wrongly classified as major traffickers. Also, due to inadequately developed management systems, 'BNDD did not know how many major traffickers were immobilized as a result of the systems approach nor how many were immobilized while the systems approach was operating. Therefore it could not find out the approach's strengths and weaknesses' (*ibid.*: 12).

The Comptroller General's conclusion was that the main effect of the operation had been disruptive of the market rather than successful in immobilising major traffickers.

> Although BNDD arrested many traffickers, temporarily dis-
> rupted the illicit activities of the . . . system and decreased
> the amount of heroin available, many major traffickers were
> still considered by BNDD to be operating as of July 1972.
>
> (*ibid.*: 2)

The shortcomings of the systems approach led to the establishment by the DEA of a rather more sophisticated Geographic-Drug Enforcement Program (G-DEP) in 1972. G-DEP is designed as an aid to the DEA's focus on major traffickers and classifies traffickers into four classes. Classification is determined by quantity or amounts being dealt, quality (the position of an individual within the trafficking network), the type of drug, the location of the violator and the type of investigation (US General Accounting Office 1984: 4). However, the General Accounting Office (1984: 4) found that the DEA's criteria for classifying who is a major trafficker were very broad; those marked down as Class I violators were often not individuals who were at the top of drug organisations.

Such approaches seem to be weak in principle and in practice. In principle, there is an assumption that there are key organisational heads who are at the centre of everything an organisation does and can do. This is close to the film demonology of 'The Godfather' but, if we pursue that analogy, we remember that in the case of the mafia there is always a new Godfather ready to succeed to the throne. Accordingly, one limitation of this approach is that

> the 'big connections' and 'top dealers' who indeed exist and who generally are not users, are in many ways the least important part of the heroin market system, because they are the most easily replaced. A new 'connection' arises for everyone put out of business.
>
> (Wilson 1985: 212; cf Trojanowicz 1990: 16)

In practice, the disappointing finding has been that 'immobilising organisations' has simply not been a very effective method of law enforcement (US General Accounting Office 1984). As Reuter and Haaga conclude

> Ease of entry [to drug trafficking as a profession] . . . lessens any hope one might have that the removal of the more experienced individuals could make a significant difference. Lower-level dealers are higher-level dealers in training. This lack of differentiation in the population suggests that incarcerating or otherwise incapacitating even a large number of experienced higher-level dealers would not seriously disrupt the markets.
>
> (Reuter and Haaga 1989: 56)

Nevertheless, the aim of incarcerating major traffickers remains central to the operations of drug enforcement agencies world-wide.

Some British examples

As the UK government's official drug misuse policy document notes

> Police action against drug traffickers is organised on three broad
> levels. At the top there are the nine Regional Crime Squads
> [RCSs] in England and Wales and the Scottish Crime Squad
> dealing with major traffickers.
>
> (Home Office 1990b: 12)

The 'drugs wings' of the RCSs were established from the recommendations of the Broome Report (partially reproduced in
the Appendix). There are seventeen drugs wings in the nine RCSs
in England and Wales (but excluding London) employing 229
officers, with a further seventy-one posts allocated by 1990/91. The
three Scottish drugs wings employ thirty-one officers with another
three posts allocated by 1990/91. In London the equivalent role
falls to the Metropolitan Police's Central Drugs Squad, consisting
of 110 officers (Home Office 1990b: 12); this squad is expected to
be absorbed into the RCS system in 1991.

The following paragraphs describe some operations mounted
at this level of enforcement. These cases illustrate something
of the range and variety of the work on one RCS drugs wing,
from international liaison (covering the importation/wholesaling
level of the market) through to surveillance on importers using
couriers and inland mid-level distributors, and finally to a lone
manufacturer, engaged in little more than user-dealing.

(1) In 1987 a drugs wing received information about the
importation of a large quantity of LSD destined for an upcoming
rock festival. A man called Jones was identified as the British end
of this operation and a raid on a place he was staying at in London
led to the discovery of photographs with picture patterns on them.
A test on the photographic paper showed it to be originally from the
United States. Liaison with the DEA established that this pattern
was destined to decorate LSD-impregnated paper squares. In a
subsequent surveillance operation Jones (who had been released
after the raid) was followed to the US where the combination
of an informant, a DEA infiltration operation and the RCS's
surveillance of Jones led to one of the largest hauls of LSD in
the US in recent years.

(2) In Operation Anvil an established target – Pike – was kept

under surveillance and was observed meeting with three other men – Hubert, Perry and Joyce. Perry was kitted out to go sailing in clothes thought to be appropriate to southern European countries. Perry and Hubert were observed setting sail and believed to be heading for Spain. The drugs wing alerted their liaison officer in Spain and Customs. Customs, in cooperation with French and Spanish Customs officers, attempted to follow the boat on its return from Spain. However, they lost sight of it during the night. The boat subsequently presented itself to Customs the next morning. Officers believed that the boat had docked in a local estuary at night and unloaded its cargo of cannabis, before sailing back to present itself as a new arrival in the morning. Subsequently officers kept surveillance on Perry and observed him taking possession of a pick-up truck; the RCS officers stopped him in the truck and found a consignment of several kilos of cannabis in it. Further surveillance work revealed that Pike and Joyce were having meetings with a number of people, often involving the exchange of considerable amounts of foreign currency. But there was no evidence that either of them actually ever handled the drugs themselves (they were believed to be using people like Perry and Hubert as couriers) and eventually the RCS brought conspiracy charges against nine people, involving suppliers at the London end as well.

(3) Because of their quasi-national role, Regional Crime Squads quite frequently work with HM Customs and Excise. This and the following case describe aspects of this work. In an intensive but relatively short-lived operation, an informant lead (from the Metropolitan Police Central Drugs Squad) led to the conclusion of the case within a week. The information led the RCS into a surveillance operation on a gang thought to be involved in cannabis importation. Members of the gang were followed on the motorway and a light plane was also used to keep track of their movement at this time. The RCS and Customs (who provided equipment such as night vision glasses) kept watch on a bay where a small boat came in and the gang formed a human chain to unload the boat's cargo into a van. Customs and the police then moved in, arresting people of several European nationalities.

(4) A much more difficult surveillance operation was mounted on a single individual, believed to be planning the sale of a large quantity of amphetamines and known to be very surveillance conscious. The RCS made a financial inquiry about this man but the man's wife was inadvertently tipped off at the bank and

the couple attempted to withdraw all their money. Officers were able to arrest them at the point of doing so and, having searched their house, found one real and one imitation gun as well as several kilos of amphetamine. Subsequent financial investigation found that the couple had around a quarter of a million pounds in various accounts, said to be the proceeds of trafficking.

(5) Finally, a case in which the squad came across a man with no known previous involvement in drugs or any other crime through monitoring the sales of certain chemicals usable in the manufacture of amphetamines and Ecstasy. From a routine follow-up of the sales of chemicals by a manufacturer, the RCS pursued this case as a potentially suspicious sale. They found that the man was a body-builder who used amphetamines as a stimulant. He admitted that he planned to sell this to fellow body-builders as well and that he had done this 'once or twice in the past'. His knowledge of drug manufacture had been simply acquired through the use of chemistry books from a local public library.

By our judgement at the beginning of the 1990s, hardly any senior British drug enforcement officers believed that the 'big trafficker' focus was really working. 'Hopeless', 'a losing battle', and 'running to avoid going backwards too fast' were the terms in which this strategy was discussed informally, privately and relatively openly at police conferences. No one would deny that individual operations made significant seizures or that traffickers were not apprehended and successfully prosecuted. They quite often were. But this process of attrition was insufficient to keep the market from expanding and becoming a nastier environment during the 1980s. Top-level drug enforcement is being recognised as a set of strategies that offer considerable bite but no stopping power. However, by the mid-1980s, drug enforcement had been gripped by a new enthusiasm.

FROM BIG TRAFFICKERS TO HOT MONEY

The US example

The Mr Big approach – relying upon the targeting of key individuals in criminal organisations – has became recognised as being only partially successful. It has been supplemented by strategies which are aimed at destabilising and destroying the *financial base* of criminal organisations. As Dombrink and Meeker (1986: 716) point out

> The adoption of these enterprise-based tools occurred at the same time as a shift in emphasis from pursuing a large number of moderately important drug cases to the nurturing of a lesser number of more important cases, often requiring a number of years to develop. This 'quality' versus 'quantity' development, which cuts across criminal categories (Wilson 1978), dovetails with the enterprise strategy.

This shift in emphasis has developed incrementally since 1978.

> In 1978 DEA began to stress the importance of immobilizing drug organizations by removing their financial resources. This position was incorporated into DEA's 1979 enforcement priorities in which DEA emphasized the need for a specific attack against traffickers' financial resources. DEA recognized that incarceration of the highest level violators alone was not substantially disruptive to many drug trafficking organizations and that an attack against their acquired assets was necessary.
> (US General Accounting Office 1984: 5)

If drug trafficking is the fastest growth area of international crime then, based on the findings of US and UK official committees, money laundering comes a close second. The US Senate Foreign Relations Committee (SFRC) Subcommittee on Narcotics and Terrorism defines it thus: 'Money laundering is the conversion of profits of illegal activities into financial assets which appear to have legitimate origins' (1990: 8). A generic model identifies three stages to money laundering: *placement*, which is the physical disposal of the cash; *layering*, the process of transferring funds through various accounts to disguise its origins; and *integration*, the movement of laundered funds into legitimate organisations (*ibid.*: 12 and see also DEA and RCMP 1988: 7–10; Devalle 1989: 8–9).

The 'get the assets' enterprise strategy of law enforcement has largely displaced the attrition strategy of 'get the people at the top' (Dombrink and Meeker 1986). A new stream of 'narco-cops' are said to have been created in the process, who have turned their attention from identifying and seizing assets of convicted traffickers to tracing the flows of laundered money (*The Economist* 1989: 5). The scale of money laundering is the subject of various guesstimates. The US SFRC Subcommittee on Narcotics and Terrorism (1990: 9) quotes a figure of $300 billion as an estimate of annual world-wide drug revenues, with $110 billion of that generated in the US alone (cf *The Economist* 1989: 5). In Britain, there are estimates of around £1,800 million worth of drug-related money flowing through the country (Home Affairs Committee 1989b, vol 2: 124). The main reason that money laundering is closely related to drug trafficking is because the latter is overwhelmingly a cash-based business, with payments in kind and loans being very much the exception.

Limitations to financial investigations

At the practical level, in the US law enforcement agencies have identified three barriers to an effective anti-money laundering strategy. One is the lack of coordination between the multiplicity of federal enforcement agencies and the sharing of intelligence. A second and related issue is that of cooperation between federal and state agencies. The third problem is a shortage of human resources involved in the 'labor intensive and time consuming' work of investigating suspected violations (US SFRC Subcommittee on Narcotics and Terrorism 1990: 35–40).

To date, probably the most famous laundering case has been that involving the Bank of Credit and Commerce International (BCCI). BCCI is alleged to have been used by General Noriega as well as a number of other major traffickers to launder their proceeds. BCCI officials are said to have knowingly cooperated in this exercise, thereby wilfully allowing the bank to be used to launder the proceeds of drug trafficking. For example, it is known that the bank moved at least $28 million of money around for Noriega and that it continued to move his money out of US jurisdiction even after he had been indicted. Furthermore the prosecuted incidents are said to be only a small number of the alleged cases in which BCCI has helped the laundering of criminal monies. Operation C-Chase,[6] a US Customs and FBI undercover 'sting' operation against BCCI uncovered the Noriega fund transfers (Bush 1988: 9). The undercover agents were involved in laundering up to $32 million in cash from the cocaine sales of one of the Medellin cartel (Gillard 1988). The laundering of the money by BCCI is said to have worked like this:

After collecting the up to $1 million cash, the [undercover] agents would have a local bank transfer the money to the BCCI branch in Tampa. BCCI then wired the money, via a New York bank, first to its head office in Luxembourg and then to BCCI in London. There it was converted into a certificate of deposit which was used as security for a loan made by BCCI in the Bahamas to a bogus corporation. Now the money was ready to be returned to the original account at BCCI in Tampa. From there, it would be wired to its final BCCI destination, a branch in Uruguay. It was taken in cash to Colombia. The difference between the amount of the certificate of deposit and the loan represented the bank's profit, according to investigators.

(Gillard 1988: 56)

Despite having a 'strong case' (US SFRC Subcommittee on Narcotics and Terrorism 1990: 45) against BCCI, under a plea bargain agreement at the beginning of 1990 the bank pleaded guilty and paid $14 million in drug money forfeiture. In exchange the US Attorney dropped all charges against BCCI (*ibid.*: 43–7). As the Subcommittee commented

The result [is] that the bank ended its criminal liability by paying no fine, but merely turning over the proceeds of drug trafficking to the federal government . . . the sole remaining defendants in this major money laundering case are individuals. Instead of eliciting information from these officials in order to fully examine the operations, structure and practices of the bank itself, the Justice Department can only probe the behaviour and motives of the individuals.

(*ibid.*: 43–6)

None the less the reverberations of the BCCI case have been greatest upon the banks, as there have been government moves delimiting bank secrecy and introducing criminal liability for bankers (for example in the case of Luxembourg, see *Police Review* 1990b: 325).

British financial policing in practice

We can look at three laundering cases within Britain.

(1) Operation Wincanton was a joint Anglo-Dutch operation, which initially involved tracking a known courier from Holland

(whose regular movements had been logged by the NDIU and Customs). The courier under the nickname of 'Red' was found to have connections in a Midlands city and was tracked (by surveillance) by a Regional Crime Squad. Customs created a profile of the types of couriers thought to be likely to be working for this organisation and successfully intercepted three couriers. The courier 'Red' was observed associating with a local small-scale entrepreneur. The RCS arrested them both and found that 'Red' was in fact the banker for the organisation, not an actual drugs carrier, involved in ferrying money between Holland and Britain. For the RCS this case is a good example of successful inter-agency cooperation between them, Customs and the Netherlands police.

Nevertheless, RCS sources emphasised that financial investigations had to be seen as being integrated into more traditional methods, rather than replacing them: 'drawing a chart that reflects intelligence doesn't provide *evidence*, so you still need surveillance and follow-ups on the ground' (RCS officer). And, as the RCS and other cooperating agencies found out, the money trail can run as dry as any other aspect of evidence. In Operation Wincanton none of the agencies was able to work back to the organisers of this importation business at the Dutch end. As they concluded, 'in the end all we did was take out the middle-men for a Dutch organisation' (RCS officer).

(2) In another RCS case, a man who had recently come out of prison, after being given a four-year sentence for dealing in heroin in the early 1980s, was arrested with his brother in possession of one kilogram of heroin which they had imported. The financial investigation led the police to believe that their sister had opened several bank accounts for them, through which up to £1.5 million had moved in a two-month period. The brothers were charged with possession with intent to supply and the police were keen to charge their sister in a conspiracy case. They raided the bank and seized evidence. However, the police were advised by the Crown Prosecution Service that the sister could not be prosecuted because it could not be proven that the money in her accounts came from her brothers and was related to their trafficking activities.

(3) A third case was prompted by the arrest of a British man in the US with fifty kilos of cocaine for which he was sentenced to twenty-two years' imprisonment. Financial investigation at the British end led drug squad officers to the man's ex-wife, believed to have been acting as his financial agent. They operated joint bank

accounts which had substantial amounts of US dollars in them, which she unsuccessfully tried to move to Switzerland just before her arrest. She was bailed and subsequently disappeared. For the drug squad, all that is left are restraint orders on the money and on the sale of an expensive house owned by her. While it is empty the house deteriorates and its financial value drops accordingly, but without a defendant in a court case the police have no option but to leave matters as they stand.

Developments in financial policing

Money laundering and the move to attacking the financial base of criminal organisations involved in drug trafficking is still a relatively new area in law enforcement. It has prompted much speculation about the amount of money said to be 'washing' its way around the international banking system; and it has also opened up new avenues in enforcement and legislative options. The emphasis upon 'the money trail' faces considerable difficulties when faced with the so-called 'ethnic' banking systems (Devalle 1989). 'Hawala' banking is said to be one means of transferring money between individuals, involving cash transfers without the use of any documentation.

Transaction receipts can be as simple as a bus ticket or a card torn in half; by presenting a matching half of such a commonplace and hardly incriminating object, a person qualifies for payment in another country. Such systems remove any need to move funds through the international banking system. The same system is said to be known as 'chiti banking' in Asia, 'chop shop banking' in China and as 'stash house' in the US and Latin America (*ICPR* 1989: 28; Devalle 1989: 9). Other techniques, which are particularly attractive to legitimate businesses 'sidelining' in drugs (see Chapter 2) or to criminal organisations possessing 'front organisations', revolve around false invoicing, payment for non-existent goods, payment several times the real worth of goods delivered, operating foreign currency exchange bureaux, and so on.

The turn towards financial policing has yet to be fully assessed. In Britain, 'chasing the money' has followed US legislation and practice as well as the general pursuance of international mutual legal assistance treaties. American officials found that, as the US has tightened up on money laundering, criminal organisations simply moved their money 'offshore' (another example of enforcement leading to displacement). This 'international loophole' has included not just the predictable financial havens, but Britain and Canada have also been cited (see DEA and RCMP 1988: 11–14). Indeed, Britain's National Drugs Intelligence Unit, in a memorandum to the Home Affairs Committee, said that 'there must be a vast amount of money circulating within the legitimate banking system that is drug-related' (NDIU 1989: 116). The NDIU's coordinator said in evidence that 'We should not forget that the United Kingdom is regarded by the United States, Canada and some others as an offshore banking system' (Home Affairs Committee 1989b, vol 2: 124). This has been the background to the development of international cooperation in order to limit the possibility of exploiting such loopholes. The international momentum has been quickened by the United Nations Convention against Illicit Traffic in Narcotic Drugs and Psychotropic Substances which removes bank secrecy as a reason for refusing to divulge information about narcotics activity and obliges signatories to make laundering a criminal and extraditable offence (US SFRC Subcommittee on Narcotics and Terrorism 1990: 56–9; *The Economist* 1989: 5).

Money laundering now seems to have become a fertile new area for legislative developments with the Home Affairs Committee (1989b: xix–xx) recommending that the Bank of England should examine any legislative developments required to counter it. However, in its response the government stated that its priority was to make the existing legislation work and to ensure bank compliance with the provisions of the existing agreements (Home Office 1990e: 9). The British government is very active in international forums (Home Office 1990e: 9), supporting for example European Commission proposals for a harmonised approach within the European Community to make money laundering a criminal offence and require banks to identify customers and ascertain on whose behalf an account is being operated (*Police Review* 1990c: 429).

So far we have described some of the main aspects of enforcement strategies targeting 'big traffickers', noting that although surveillance, undercover work, attempts to immobilise trafficking organisations and financial investigations all add up to a formidable arsenal in bringing individuals to book, the trade goes on. A recent response to this, to be explored in the following chapters, is to re-emphasise the middle and lower levels of drug enforcement. However, we conclude the saga of the search for the big traffickers with one further possibility, difficult to put into practice, but intriguing in its implications.

Randomisation: a practical proposal?

One of the annoying things about drug enforcement, when viewed from the perspective of the enforcers, is that traffickers (or at least some of them) become adept at working out current enforcement strategies, and developing counter-strategies. Throughout this study, we emphasise the tendency for traffickers to keep their organisations small and flexible, an understandable response to enforcement that for several decades announced its commitment to immobilising large organisations. More recently, as we shall describe in Chapter 7, there has been increasing stress on policing down market, and in turn this will prompt new counter-measures by traffickers.

Recently, a distinction has been drawn between 'novice' and 'experienced' smugglers at the importation level (Reuter *et al.* 1988). The significance of this distinction becomes clearer when considering what are called 'modelling adaptations' made by smugglers. At its simplest this means that smugglers employ 'least-risk' routes of importation. As the risk of a particular route increases (or is perceived to have increased) perhaps due to more seizures, enhanced law enforcement, uncovering of particular methods of importation, etc., smugglers will adapt by changing the routes, amounts or methods they employ. This, in other words, is a restatement of the proposition that drug markets and law enforcement continuously interact and shape one another. In Reuter *et al.*'s (1988) terms, smugglers 'learn by doing', and this experience-based model guides future behaviour.

> This view of smuggler learning and adaptation can be more generally applied to drug enforcement at all levels. There is a parallel between the border crossing 'learning by doing' cycle and drug enforcement at the street level. Local police officials have described a specific situation where the formation of a new undercover task force began to increase arrests and convictions. After a period of 18 months, the dealers developed a complex system of lieutenants, holders, runners, and money men to

insulate themselves from prosecution. It then took the police almost two years to identify and separate the components of the new network and adjust their own operations accordingly.

(Reuter *et al.* 1988: 120)

So the general dilemma faced by enforcement agencies is that familiarity with their methods by smugglers actually makes the smuggler potentially more adept at circumventing those methods. One potential counter-strategy available to enforcement could be that there should be no *general* enforcement strategy. If enforcement strategies are randomised to become less predictable, then traffickers would be less able to develop counter-measures.

What might this mean in practice? This is difficult to imagine. Reuter *et al.*'s (1988) study looked at the effects of increased interdiction efforts at the US borders and argued that it has had limited effects on the retail price (and availability) of drugs.[7] We do not need to look into the reasons for this here. The important point is that having argued that smugglers learn and adapt from the pattens of law enforcement, the obvious implication must be that the more predictable law enforcement efforts are, the less successful they are likely to be in the long run against experienced traffickers. Within these parameters Reuter *et al.* recommend that law enforcement strategies should be randomised, to create maximum uncertainty in the market.

> Random allocation can greatly increase the impact of additional interdiction resources. Smugglers can adapt efficiently only when they can form good estimates of the interdiction rates associated with particular routes. If they know that three routes will have higher interdiction rates, but they do not know which three they are, the adaptation will be relatively ineffective.
>
> (*ibid.*: 107)

One of the present authors initially responded to the randomisation proposal as a 'strategy of despair' (Dorn 1989) but, on reflection, it is difficult to see quite what other conclusion results from an application of a model of drug trafficking as being in interaction with and learning from law enforcement agencies. Certainly its implications have not been tried out. But practical problems would arise if it were attempted. Randomisation would be expensive to enforcement agencies, who employ routines at least partly on the grounds of economy. There would also be costs in terms of agents' familiarity with particular locations and that of moving staff and equipment around (Reuter *et al*. 1988: 121). Also, as Manning (1980: 141) suggests, detectives work in particular ways partly because they have never been trained to work in any other way. It is doubtful if organisational coherence, direction or goals could be maintained if enforcement agencies seriously tried to vary their operations in unpredictable ways. The result might be rather chaotic.

By comparison, trafficking organisations are small and flexible enough to change their strategies rapidly, without disintegrating. From any serious perspective, the ambition to locate and immobilise the big traffickers faces serious difficulties. One response to this is to change one's views of what constitutes a priority target.

Chapter 6

City drug squads
Surveillance and buy operations

British drug enforcement is organised into three levels, each of which is intended to target a corresponding level of the drug market. In this chapter we present some material on the middle-level response – the level of county and city police drug squads and, within London, Area Drug Squads. The rationale for targeting this level is that if there is a chain of supply within the market from importer through to wholesalers and retailers, then it makes sense to tackle the middle of the market, since this is the conduit between the two ends of the market.

> Drug wholesalers represent a vital and enduring link in the capacities of drug networks to continuously supply their customers, often in the face of strong enforcement pressure. Resources devoted to eliminating the more careful and cautious offenders might well cause market interruptions, with difficulties in replacing sanctioned wholesalers with comparably efficient dealers . . . improved police allocation of narcotics investigative resources might make promotion or recruitment of replacement wholesalers more expensive and hazardous, thereby constraining the movements of more active dealers.
>
> (PERF 1986: 12)

In Britain the middle level is the province of the specialist drug squads in each police force. The government's strategy document says that, 'The strength of police force drug squads in England and Wales, in 1989, at some 880 officers, was more than 40% higher than at the end of 1983' (Home Office 1990b: 12). As we described in Chapter 5 the 'top' level of the market falls to the RCSs. The theory is that the RCSs are supposed only to investigate major crimes which cut across the boundaries of county forces, but in practice the RCSs in some 'quieter areas' are used as an adjunct to the work of a county force, investigating serious crime within the boundaries of a single force (Darbyshire 1990: 19). It should be remembered that the organisational levels or 'tiers' of enforcement do not correspond in any neat or easy way to distinctions in the market. In practice, deciding which targets 'belong' to which enforcement level can be problematic.

A METROPOLITAN AREA DRUG SQUAD: FOCUS ON SURVEILLANCE

By far the greatest amount of drug activity and arrests take place within the Metropolitan Police region. The Metropolitan Police Central Drugs Squad is analogous to an RCS drugs wing. Below that, responsibility for dealing with the perceived 'middle' of the market falls to the eight Area Drug Squads in the Met. The purpose of the Area Drug Squads is summed up in their terms of reference:

> The object of the Area Drug Squad shall be the arrest and prosecution of persons engaged in the illegal supplying of controlled drugs . . . whose method of operation, either by virtue of expertise or geographical field of activities is beyond the capabilities of Divisional resources.

A squad is headed by an inspector and will generally consist of about thirteen officers, working in three or four teams and reporting to an area Chief Superintendent. The squads will usually work closely with an Asset Confiscation Desk (formerly Financial Investigation Team) responsible for financial investigations under the Drug Trafficking Offences Act 1986. With the extension of asset confiscation to other categories of crime, the financial investigators also work on cases under the provisions of the Criminal Justice Act 1988 (which authorises asset confiscation for crimes if the defendants can be found to have profited by more than £10,000) and the Prevention of Terrorism Act 1989.

In one Area Drug Squad we found that the priorities, targets and methods tend to be set by a combination of the views of the head of the squad, the individuals making up the squad and a conception of the nature of the 'drug milieu' which they perceived to be representative of their area. The middle level of the market was defined by this squad in terms of the level of the criminal organisation and the amounts, usually multi-kilo, being traded.[8]

But – reflecting something of the fluid and changing nature of the drug market – the squad also found itself running across and sometimes targeting relative 'newcomers' to the market.

The cases described below involved surveillance techniques, both static and mobile. The squad, however, employed a wider range of methods than those described including telephone surveillance, undercover operations and joint work with Customs and other police forces.

Case study: from London to Scotland

This case involved a Scottish family of 'career criminals' who were well known to the police. The Worthingtons had moved down from Scotland and settled in London in the early 1970s, while other members of their large family were spread about the country. A working-class family from an estate in Glasgow, they settled on an estate in London and were described as 'inbred, pretty incestuous really' (drug squad officer). The Worthingtons had become fairly well established as small-scale dealers in amphetamine sulphate, and to a lesser extent in cocaine and heroin; they had no other known source of legitimate income, although painting and decorating was mentioned as a possible business outlet. A tip-off to the Area Drug Squad from an informant led to a surveillance operation on the family. The drug squad established as the 'main target' George Worthington, the head of the family (who had previous convictions for robbery and armed robbery). Because they had no sophisticated anti-surveillance measures they could be followed with relative ease. The surveillance work established that the informant's tip-off was correct: the family were involved in running drugs between Scotland and London, but establishing evidence proved to be more difficult because the family used up to five or six different addresses which made keeping watch on all of them impossible.

This was a profitable operation for the Worthingtons and they engaged in conspicuous consumption of their proceeds. One officer said that unless they were working they would be 'in the pub for the duration' sometimes flashing a wallet with a wad of up to £2,000 in it. But it may have been that it was precisely this lifestyle which brought about their downfall. On a train the family drank too much and were warned for loud and yobbish behaviour. The British Transport Police (BTP) were notified and arrested them. They were found to be carrying a small amount of drugs.

The Worthingtons also had £1,600 in cash on them which they were unable to explain. The BTP notified the Met and the case was effectively closed. Up to ten of the family stood trial for conspiracy in connection with the possession and supply of cocaine and amphetamines.

The Worthingtons were a family of criminal diversifiers. In the eyes of the police, they were seen to be middle-market dealers – by virtue of the amounts they were working with (a few kilograms) and because their business crossed police force boundaries. None the less, despite their precaution of using several addresses they were relatively unsophisticated and effectively tripped themselves up; their capture involved little detective policing.

Case study: from a small dealer to a large conspiracy

In a 1988 importation operation the squad liaised with Customs and European police through Interpol. An informant said to the squad that a man called Edwards had access to between four and six ounces of cocaine which he was going to collect from what the police call 'a known drugs address' and would then sell it onto someone dealing in larger quantities than Edwards did. Edwards had a long history of involvement in the drug trade (both using and dealing) and was said to be trusted by a number of different organisations, without actually directly being a member of any one of them. However, the cocaine deal fell through when Edwards refused to work with the rather disorganised suppliers.

> It turned out that the cocaine inquiry collapsed because he didn't like the attitude of the people he was dealing with. He said they were mad. He said they were absolutely ludicrous the way they were behaving. They were taking drugs and dealing in them and didn't know what they were doing half the time, so he stepped out of that one.
>
> (drug squad officer)

But having already identified Edwards as an operator in the market, the drug squad continued its surveillance operation on him. Edwards was subsequently approached by a man who said he needed someone to go to Spain to arrange a cannabis importation. Edwards and Walker (also a man with previous drugs convictions) flew out to Spain. The surveillance operation on them continued while they were out in Spain as two officers from the drug squad also travelled out. There they observed Edwards and Walker meeting a man; subsequently twenty-six kilograms of cannabis resin was delivered to their hotel. The drugs were left with a third man who smuggled them into Britain using a boat. Through their surveillance operation on Edwards the drug squad had already established that he had a safe flat, close to his own address. The police kept watch on both premises. A woman went to the safe flat and after leaving the premises was arrested with about four kilos of the cannabis, which confirmed that the drugs were in the safe flat. Subsequently they watched Edwards go to the safe flat and return with a holdall. A raid on Edwards' address and the safe flat led to the seizure of the cannabis, the link between them further confirmed by the packaging: both were 'wrapped in exactly in the same way, same gear, so provable it's untrue' (drug squad officer).

This case, like that of the Worthingtons, illustrates that traffickers moving quite large amounts of drugs are not necessarily very sophisticated. Enforcement may be based on the most basic of starting points (an informant) and relatively simple (mostly static) surveillance techniques. In the words of the officer in charge of the case:

> certainly having taken it from what the informant told us, all the indicators were that we were onto something and it just developed from there . . . to my mind it is a classic example of starting off with a man who is a trusted small dealer in his own right, and moving onto a larger conspiracy.

In practice, for an Area Drug Squad the middle of the market as we have seen covers a number of possibilities from importation to intra-national operations and wholly local cases. None the less these officers sometimes see themselves as fighting a losing battle against bureaucratic and organisational constraints, failing to keep up with the technological sophistication of the most organised dealers:

> We have had for three or four years now . . . financial restrictions that are strangling our ability to work . . . certainly I find it personally very frustrating when I follow a man around for eight hours and they say 'well, you have to go back for a debrief now because you can't work overtime' . . . It is [all] down to finance. They've tried to run the police force like a business . . . between nine to five, five days a week. . . . I mean how can you work eight hours a day on this – you can't. [It] is hardly sufficient to

travel to where they [dealers from other cities] are to look at them. . . . We are investigating crime on a cut-rate basis and it is bloody ridiculous to be quite honest.

(drug squad officer)

Although we have shown them working completely outside of their force boundaries, this is still the exception for these officers. In this they see themselves as the poor relations of the RCSs:

the Regional Crime Squads can travel from here to the borders of Scotland and talk to the police forces all the way through . . . they have got the facilities and the equipment. . . . At the counties they will have a central base and the people in those offices will be from perhaps four or five different police forces. All working together, all with the same radio communications, no problems about talking to each other or overtime.

(drug squad officer)[9]

Indeed radio communication is a bane of the lives of the Area Drug Squad officers, even to the extent of working with other officers from their own force.

We can't go and work with the Central Drugs Squad, well we can, we do work together. But our radios are not compatible with theirs, so you can have twenty, forty people out working – twenty of us, twenty of them. And we all have to carry two radios each – to communicate to our own and to communicate to them. And then you get to the situation, 'well I'm sorry there ain't enough radios to go round'.

(drug squad officer)

Finally, for the Area Drug Squad there are also problems of ownership of cases, as jobs determined as being outside their terms of reference are dealt with by the Central Drugs Squad: 'We are not jealous of them. I mean good luck – get on and do the job, because personally I don't care who nicks them as long as they get nicked' (drug squad officer).

A CITY DRUG SQUAD: GOING UNDERCOVER

Undercover work is an art, not a science.

(Fuqua 1978: 181)

Undercover work, together with surveillance and financial

investigations, are methods that may be used in various combinations against a variety of targets. We have chosen to describe undercover methods in relation to the middle range of the market for two reasons. First, because the case we describe in detail here is of a middle-level target by a City Drug Squad. Second, because of the relationship between undercover and 'buy' operations. As we argue below, 'buy' operations are an interesting example of a policing method working in both 'up' and 'down' directions. It is in this middle range that the relatively sophisticated 'criminal diversifiers' are most likely to be found (see Chapter 3; Waymont and Wright 1989). These 'targets', often already known to the police in connection with crimes other than trafficking, may be surveillance-wise, resisting direct visual or electronic monitoring, and may also be relatively sophisticated in their shielding of financial aspects of their business.

This leaves open the enforcement tactic probably most feared by the career criminal – various provocations by undercover officers themselves posing as traffickers and offering to trade. There are two main undercover tactics. The first, the undercover 'buy', has a long pedigree and is utilised by enforcement agencies in most countries. The second, the undercover 'sell', occurs in the US where, although often described as a form of entrapment, it secures convictions (sometimes of public figures, who are buying for personal use rather than to re-sell) and will be discussed in Chapter 8.

Buy bust operations

The American literature is replete with examples of 'buy' operations (for example see Drug Enforcement Administration 1982: 99–112; Moore 1977: 140–7; Fuqua 1978: 181–90). In essence, the operation is a simple one; a plainclothes officer poses as a drug buyer and induces a trafficker to sell to him or her (for a history of undercover practices see Marx 1988).

> Police have used 'undercover' detectives on occasions for many years. The drug squad did not introduce the practice, but undercover work became a regular feature of their specialised duties. If detectives wanted to work under cover in a pub, a popular meeting place, or indeed, in a hippie community, they had to remain inconspicuous by donning the same casual clothing as their suspects. Gradually, permanent undercover

operations became established . . . the disguised detective has
to be an actor. A good actor becomes identified with the role he
is playing, casting his own personality aside.

(Pritchard and Laxton 1978: 27)

Themes of dangerousness and excitement are never very far
away in descriptions of undercover work. Thus Fuqua's list
of qualities needed for undercover work is desire to do the
job, self-confidence, resourcefulness, courage, adaptability and
incorruptibility (1978: 181–2). And one regular recurring
feature is the need to maintain a convincing 'face', to be able
to play the role of a drug user or of a potential drug buyer
convincingly (Skolnick 1966; Fuqua 1978; Pritchard and Laxton
1978; Drug Enforcement Administration 1982; Lyman 1987). If
narcotics policing 'emphasize[s] the craftsmanlike possibilities of
policework' (Skolnick 1966: 138) and 'gives the policeman an
especially interesting, gamelike kind of job' (*ibid.*: 117), then it
would seem that undercover work is a particular representation of
this. Beneath the fantasy however there may well be a messy world
which commands less attention when the story is related after the
event.

There is a distinction between two levels of immersion in the
undercover role. The plainclothes officer 'working the street' for
a typical shift is doing 'partial undercover' work, becoming only
marginally involved in a local drug scene. In contrast, 'deep
undercover' work is a full-time activity (Pistone and Woodley
1988).

The agent adopts an identity and lifestyle that is maintained on
a 24-hour basis for a lengthy period of time. . . . Infrequent
and clandestine contacts are made with fellow agents during
this period of complete submersion in the drug subculture.

(Williams and Guess 1981: 236)

Making the connection

Here we describe a case study of one officer on a deep undercover
operation. (The targets in this operation are described as the
Bennetts and the Morgans in Chapter 3.) The background is that
a drug squad was working on a strategy of posing as potential buyers
of amphetamine with the eventual aim – not successful as it turned
out – of 'working up' to the point of production at the factory.

In this case an informant's tip led to an operation in which officers went undercover, posing as potential drug buyers. One of the officers – Trevor – played the main role, doing the negotiating and the exchange. For the undercover officer, entry into the market initially relied on an informant[10] who duped a minor dealer into introducing the officer to a key intermediary or link man (or 'maker of introductions'). This link man, called Henry and described as a 'Mr Fixit', was himself involved in supplying amphetamine.[11] Trevor, the undercover officer, was introduced as a man interested in doing some business, in this case purchasing multi-kilos of amphetamine.

Apparently satisfied with Trevor's bona fides, Henry willingly offered himself as a man who could make the necessary connections. Through Henry, Trevor was introduced to Malcolm Bennett, a young man within a family of career criminals, whose 'dad took him on meets with good villains' (drug squad officer). This family business consisted of the son (Malcolm) and his father, with the son acting as a runner for his father, a former bank robber who had only recently come out of prison after receiving a fourteen-year sentence for a bank robbery.

> The son is controlled by his father, the son does the negotiating, does the selling on the instructions of his father. . . . He [the father] was shrewd, he used his own son to take all the risks . . . [so although] we arrested him, we interviewed him, he had been there, seen it . . . and everything . . . he has never been charged.
> (drug squad officer)

Malcolm met with Trevor and sold one kilogram of amphetamine for £2,500 as a form of 'test purchase'. Trevor made it clear that he was interested in purchasing a lot more and they agreed that another five kilos would be supplied by Malcolm. But in between these two deals, Malcolm being, according to the drug squad officer, 'a bit of a gobby sod' started 'shouting his mouth off' in public about how he was now involved in big business and that he had a big buyer. This proved to be valuable for the police because it enabled Trevor to go back to his intermediary, Henry, saying that he was unhappy since Malcolm's loud behaviour was obviously attracting attention to him as the 'big buyer' as well. Without actually pulling out of the deal already arranged with Malcolm – the officer in charge said the police 'being a bit greedy' decided to pursue all possible purchases – Trevor asked Henry about other potential sources of supply. Henry then effected another introduction, this time by giving Trevor's telephone number to another intermediary from a separate team. It is this transaction which we describe in detail.

Arranging a buy

Having given his telephone number to Henry, Trevor was then contacted by Dave. Dave acted as the 'runner' for the second team, conducting all the preliminary face-to-face negotiations with Trevor. The two other men in this team appeared only once, at the time of the exchange itself. Dave telephoned Trevor on a Sunday saying, 'I understand you're interested in a deal. . . . I can do as much you want, but I don't like talking on the phone'. They arranged to meet the next day at 7.00 p.m. The version given here is the one recounted in court describing the arrangements for the deal and the exchange. Trevor did not use a concealed tape recorder, because of the risk of being found out. Instead the various meetings were recorded as notes from his memory of the conversations. None the less, the details were not disputed in court by Dave's defence.[12]

Although a 'test purchase' had been required from the Bennetts the advantage of being in the field posing as a potential buyer meant that Trevor had already established his bona fides.

> Word had got through to the second team that 'yes your street cred is very good because we know that you have already purchased a kilo from the other firm who we happen to know anyway'. There was a link but not a criminal link. . . . So they didn't require a test purchase to get the credibility of the purchaser.
>
> (drug squad officer)

The first meeting took place at a pub. Trevor arrived on time, bought himself a drink and waited by the bar. Dave arrived some ten to fifteen minutes late and went up to him at the bar saying, 'Are you Trevor? Hello, I'm Dave'. Trevor replied 'Thank fuck you've arrived. I thought it was a fucking wind up'. After buying drinks they went and sat down at a table. Trevor's notes recorded the substance of their conversation as being:

Dave: How much do you want?

Trev: Five k.

Dave: All right, but I'll have to speak to my partner . . . so all we've got to do is sort out what gear you want.

Trev: What's the difference?

Dave explained that there are two different prices available per kilo because they were of different levels of purity. The higher priced 'gear [had] only been jumped on once' (i.e. only been cut with other substances once).

Trev: It's that good, is it?

Dave: It's not pure, but it's good stuff, fucking good.

Trevor plumped for the cheaper stuff, which Dave was offering for £2,200 per kilo. Having established the amount and its availability, Trevor tried to negotiate the price down a bit.

Trev: You can't come down a bit, can you?

Dave: How much are you talking about?

Trev: Well if you come down to two's [£2,000 per kilo], we could make a monkey [£500] each.

Dave: I can't come down.

Trev: I'll tell my man we're dealing at two three [£2,300 per kilo] and if you back me up I'll have a drink with you later.

Trevor is himself posing as the employee or 'front' man for a buyer for whom he is working. By trying to negotiate the price and asking Dave to 'back him up' in any questions about the price at which they are trading, Trevor tries to bolster his identity as a crook and to dispel any suspicions that he might be anything else. Dave agreed that he would help Trevor to make some money 'on the side' by not disputing the higher figure of £2,300 per kilo which Trevor would quote as the price at which the deal was being made.

They then moved onto the arrangements for the exchange. Trevor pointed out that Dave had got his telephone number, but that he (Trevor) could not contact Dave. Dave did not want to give out a telephone number saying, 'I don't know you and you don't know me.'

Trev: You're mucking me about again.

Dave: No, I'm not mucking you about, but you've got to be careful in this business.

They left the pub after agreeing that Dave would telephone Trevor on the next day (Tuesday) to arrange the exchange for the day after (Wednesday). Dave failed to call on Tuesday and in fact phoned on Wednesday morning, apologising for not calling before. Trevor was angry about this and said, 'I'm not going to arrange with you if you're not going to turn up'. Under pressure because of his failure to hold up his side of the arrangements, Dave then agreed to give Trevor his telephone number. Unexpectedly Dave called Trevor again in the evening of the same day, and asked for another meeting, saying 'I've got a couple of samples for you'. Trevor agreed, saying 'All right, [but] you're a pest'. They arranged to meet at another pub in that evening. At the second meeting, the record of their conversation as presented in court was as follows.

Trev: What's all this about?
Dave: We've got to sort it out and arrange what gear you want.
Trev: I can't understand why it's urgent.
Dave: I don't know what gear you want.
Trev: I've already told you.

Dave had brought along two samples of amphetamine of different purities for Trevor to try, so that he could choose which one he wanted to buy. Trevor leant towards Dave, who slipped the two small packets inside Trevor's T-shirt. Trevor went to the toilet where he inspected the two packets. He came back pretending to have sampled the contents saying, 'I shouldn't have tried them both'. Dave replied, 'I know, I've never had so much speed in one go before'.[13] After confirming which one he wanted they move on to discuss the details of the exchange.

Dave: Are you sure the money's there?
Trev: Yes.

Dave accounted for his concern about the arrangements on the grounds that 'these are really bad people I'm working with'. Finally Dave said 'I'll call tonight, if it's on I'll say "tell Trev to phone Dave", if not I'll say "tell Trev Dave phoned".'

They agreed that the exchange would be on the Friday, arranging to meet at lunchtime in the same pub where Trevor and Dave had had their first meeting.

The bust goes a bit wrong

On Friday Trevor went to the pub and shortly afterwards he was approached by Dave, who greeted him, saying 'Hello Trev, what's happening?' Trev replied, 'Sweet FA.' Dave asked to see the money and Trevor made a call on a portable phone to call it in. A second undercover officer drove into the car park and Trevor and Dave got into the car.

> Trev: The money's in the briefcase [chained to wrist of other officer], if it's a rip you get covered in diamond smoke' [i.e. opening the briefcase would let out a dye].

Another officer said,

> We called in the flash money . . . they viewed the money and counted it . . . the money was then sent away again. In fact from then on in, the money never appeared again because we have strict rules that the money and the drugs never come together. . . . That money would never ever come back in, obviously in case there is a rip-off.
>
> (drug squad officer)

Although this explanation is couched primarily in terms of the security of the money, here as elsewhere in the undercover operation the police are following the 'rules of the game'. Obviously posing as real drug buyers they have to seek to play the role as realistically as possible. Their understanding of drug operations is that the money and the drugs are never together at the same time, but exchanged separately, either in different places at the same time or at different times. Their security concerns dovetail with the usual way in which the market operates.

At this point Garry[14] came into the picture and took over the operation. He walked into the pub and said to Trevor words to the effect that 'I am the main man, I am the man you are actually dealing with, the other guy [Dave], he is just my runner'. There then ensued an argument between Garry and Dave, the former being angry with Dave for giving Trevor his phone number and apparently for not keeping Garry adequately informed. Garry said 'Why didn't you tell us his number, with our contacts we could have checked him out'.

The three of them left the pub and walked down the road, during which time Colin had driven into the car park and left the car with the drugs in it. Garry said that he was willing to continue the deal and they went back to the pub. Garry then left the scene and was followed by other officers. In the pub, Dave said that the gear was in the car and that after Trevor had inspected it, he could call in the money (again) and the exchange would proceed. They went to the car and got in, Dave in the driver's seat with Trevor in the passenger seat. Reaching behind his seat Dave got out a plastic bag. Trevor examined it and confirmed that it was amphetamine.

Trevor then made another call, apparently to call in the money. In fact, the call acted as a pre-arranged signal for other officers in the vicinity to 'attack the car'. Trevor, still playing his role, escaped by running away and, in the course of doing so, headbutted another officer. 'We obviously had to make it look good' (drug squad officer). Dave was arrested there and Garry was arrested later at his home. Colin was arrested much later:

> We lost him, we couldn't find him anywhere. In fact we arrested him two or three weeks later. [It] had to be an armed operation because of the knowledge that we had, we knew that he was an absolute[ly] crazy man. We took him out.
>
> (drug squad officer)

Target number two gets cold feet

After running away from the scene of Dave's arrest, Trevor then 'called' on his purchase of another five kilos from the Bennetts by making a phone call to Malcolm. According to the drug squad officer, 'It becomes quite apparent from that phone call that things are not right'. This cannot have been due to any communication between the two teams since 'We were that quick there was no communication between the one group and the other group'.

So what happened? According to the drug squad officer

> They [the Bennetts] had a council of war the night before [the day of the deal], and they were not happy that a man would pay £2,500 for a kilo of gear that wasn't as strong as they had said. I mean they told him [Trevor] that it was that strong that he could jump on it several times and still be able to sell it on the streets. In fact it could have been jumped on maybe twice at a push. So it was weak for a dealer's quantity. It wasn't weak compared to the

street stuff, but it was weak from a dealer's point of view. So they came to the conclusion that it was a rip off. . . . [They thought] it was a team of villains who were going to rip their five kilos off. So when the phone call went in to them, they said 'What we need is a little more credibility from you, we have never heard of you, we are not really happy at this stage. Can you give us a reference?' . . . That incidentally can be done.

However, at this stage the undercover operation was discontinued and the drug squad moved in to arrest all the participants.

[But] in the end it was an executive decision to end it. We decided it would be too dangerous, we decided that the risk would be too great . . . although it had all looked very good when the undercover officer escaped, it did look good.

(drug squad officer)

Malcolm and Henry were arrested and charged with supplying the first kilogram of amphetamine. Both were sentenced to fifteen months' imprisonment each for conspiracy to supply, on the basis of supplying half a kilo each and as supposedly their first involvement in supplying. Although the one kilo was merely a 'taster' for a much larger deal, the judge took no account of this. One officer describes this sentence as 'atrocious', the judge being very lenient indeed. The decision in this case had a bearing on Dave's trial as well. The judge there said he was thinking of a sentence of four years, but took into account the sentence in the case of Malcolm and Henry. Dave was sentenced to two years' imprisonment and had £1,000 in assets confiscated.

Appraisal of buy operations

Although 'buy bust' itself is the most well-known technique there are in fact a number of related operations which come under the general heading of 'buy operations' (cf Lyman 1987: 104–7). Such operations are essentially part of undercover police work, involving officers making buys themselves or keeping surveillance on a buy made by an informant (see Chapter 8). In the large US literature the former is called the 'agent buy' and the latter the controlled 'informant buy' (Drug Enforcement Administration 1982: 100). Informants making supervised buys could be seeking to establish that a suspected person is a seller, possibly with a plan of making more buys and to 'introduce' an undercover officer as another buyer later. The more complex uses of an informant buy are a means of gathering intelligence about the market and some people operating within it. The use of such participating informants (see Chapter 8) is said to be strictly controlled, but under such circumstances, informants are allowed to possess controlled drugs. However, as this drug squad officer makes clear, such 'protection' has its limitations.

> We make it plain to them from the outset [that] the only time they [informants] can ever have drugs in their possession is if we tell them to and, although they don't know it, we have actually got permission from a very high level that they can have their £5 worth of cannabis on them as a sample they just purchased. They know it and I tell them, I tell all my informants outright: if you ever bleep me or ring me up and say that 'I have just been nicked and I had ten deals in my pocket, come and get me out of it', I shall come down there and say hammer this bastard into the ground and take him to court and send him to prison forever. And they [informants] know it upfront. That is the first thing that I always say to an informant when he is going to work for me.
>
> (drug squad officer)

Agent buys can also be subdivided into two types: the 'buy bust' itself might involve making a number of small preliminary buys from a dealer, then arranging the purchase of a much larger amount and arresting the supplier at the point of the transaction.

> The greatest advantage of the buy/bust is that it is economical. It allows the unit to make arrests for major sales while expending funds for only one or two small preliminary buys.
>
> (Drug Enforcement Administration 1982: 101)

An arrest does not always need to be made on the spot and there is also the 'walk-away buy', where after an officer has made a buy an arrest warrant is obtained subsequently. This has the advantages of protecting the identity of the undercover officer or informant making the buy and permits a number of raids in an area to be coordinated. There are also disadvantages:

transient dealers may have moved on and the co-ordination of simultaneous raids is expensive in police resource terms (*ibid.*: 101).

Implicit in the DEA's vision of buy bust operations are both the idea of 'working up the chain' or 'buying up the ladder' (Moore 1977: 22) from street dealers to retailers and wholesalers and the aim of clearing locales identified as drug-dealing locations. But the strategy of working toward making bigger busts contains other dangers too.

> The central metaphor in buy-bust is escalation, because one wants to make larger buys from a dealer larger than the person from whom the first buys are made, one hopes to involve larger and larger amounts of cash, and thus the risk to all parties increases. Agents are worried because the money might be ripped off, and drug dealers are worried about their drugs being ripped off as well. Both groups carry weapons into such scenes. Both distrust the other. Like other kinds of enforcement, the higher the risk the higher the gain, but the greater the loss if something goes wrong. It very often does.
>
> (Manning 1980: 175)

But escalation, or seeking to make larger buys, has proved to be a tactic of limited utility in drug enforcement, particularly in catching higher-level dealers.

> Through the years, the domestic drug law enforcement effort has been criticized for engaging too frequently in investigations of a short term transactional nature – commonly referred to as 'buy bust' cases. . . . In November 1981, the Attorney General's Committee on DEA–FBI Coordination noted that DEA has viewed drug cases as transactional in nature and has made limited use of the more sophisticated techniques which are essential to the successful investigation of large, complex criminal organizations. . . . Recognizing that 'buy bust' investigative techniques lack direct results against top-level traffickers, DEA has reduced the use of this investigative approach.
>
> (US General Accounting Office 1984: 24–5)

And commenting on the impact of this method on local drug markets Eck (1989b: 9) says

Though this has been a standard tactic for years, there is no evidence that these investigations result in more than a temporary decline in drug availability. Further, removing a local dealer can precipitate violence, as groups of traffickers fight for the newly available market.

Buy bust strategies have a curious and uncertain position in Britain. Although undercover buys of the type we have described in this chapter do occur, there remain potential sensitivities because of the agent provocateur aspect. In considering this issue the Home Affairs Committee (1989b: xxix) opined

We are not convinced that the drugs problem can be tackled entirely by traditional methods of law enforcement . . . changes would be considered only as a response to the exceptional circumstances of the drugs threat and would require strict safeguards in order to function effectively and satisfy a court of law.

Even more controversial are the types of bust operations which members of the Home Affairs Committee observed in Washington, DC. We look at such 'stings' and 'sell operations' in Chapter 8 in discussing sensitive issues in policing. If such techniques were to become a part of policing drug markets in Britain, it would reflect a tendency for policing in the 1990s to move 'down market'.

Chapter 7

Policing localities
Street operations

'Demand reduction' entered the vocabulary of drug policy in a big way from 1989 onwards. Its increasing use reflects the realisation that whatever is done to stop traffickers at the upper and middle levels of the market, large quantities will continue to get through to the lower levels of the market.[15]

What are the prospects of suppressing the trade by countering the retail trade in its various forms, or by discouraging potential consumers from purchasing drugs, or by emphasising the punitive response to all consumers with the intention of scaring them away from drugs or into treatment programmes? Demand reduction can mean any or all of these things, depending upon who is using the term and with what intent. This chapter examines enforcement strategies at this level of the market – especially at the seller–consumer interface.

TARGETING SELECT AREAS

Retail or local drug markets often inhabit particular areas or locales. The most public of such locations sometimes become synonymous with drug dealing, and attract intensive police action. Essentially police activity in such areas is marked by selectivity: a street, a public house or an estate is marked out as a locale for drug dealing, which has achieved some prominence (whether local or more widespread) and possibly public complaints too. Enforcement activity against such locations does have a demonstrative aspect since the police are after all seeking to clear what have become identified as areas of public concern. Here we describe three types of selectivity. First, raids, which are perhaps the most public manifestation of targeting by the police. Second, 'sweeps', which are best described in the the US literature as the clearing of particular streets and areas, and which represent an intermediate strategy between raids and our final example. Third, we describe the targeting of a particular road through surveillance operations.

Raids

A well-known form of law enforcement is the police raid. Raids are visible and sometimes violent demonstrations of police power. In this sense they are clearly to be positioned at the crude end of police strategies.

In the late 1980s one of the two most visible targets of police raid tactics have been some areas with sizeable populations of African-Caribbean descent. Two frequent complaints have been that these are little more than 'fishing raids' (where, as with many estates, the police are bound to find some drugs) and that the police have used such raids as a substitute for regular action against dealers. More recently, these raids have been justified on the basis of being targeted against cocaine and crack.[16]

In Wolverhampton in May 1989 a raid by the West Midlands police on a pub on the Heath Town Estate led to an alleged 'riot'. Press and police accounts said that up to five hundred people had thrown bricks and petrol bombs at the police (*Police Review* 1989a: 1055; Ward 1989: 3; Bowcott 1989: 24; Hoyland 1989: 2). In fact, an investigation by the Channel 4 programme *Hard News* in June 1989 found that fewer than sixty people were actually involved. A local drug agency worker we spoke to said, 'The police have backpedalled on the size of the crowd, it's now about twenty or thirty'. And reviewing the recent history of police action around the area this agency worker pointed to the symbolic and displacement effects of raids.

> They did another pub with nowhere near as many officers. Then it moved to the Traveller's Rest and now it's probably moved somewhere else. . . . Two pubs have now been closed so it's just moved on to another place. . . . Whether [the raids] are a serious attempt to eradicate drugs I doubt, it may be they want to show they're doing their job.
>
> (interview, 1989)

In October 1989 selected media representatives were invited to observe the preparatory planning and subsequent action on the

Broadwater Farm estate in 'Operation Kingfisher' (an interestingly titled operation, given the allegations of 'fishing raids'). The main intention of such raids is to demonstrate police 'control' of a problem and an area. The type and amount of seizures are secondary criteria, although they certainly have had the potential to embarrass the police. So for example the 'crack raid' in Wolverhampton led to the seizure of minimal amounts of crack and no charges related to its discovery. In responding to allegations that 'Operation Kingfisher' was just a 'media circus' – particularly since only limited seizures and arrests were made – the Met responded by arguing that media involvement and talk had meant that dealers had been 'tipped off' and left the estate (Stern 1989: 2,070–1; Grannatt 1989: 2,124–5; Caseby, 1989: 4).

The second main target of police raids arose during the summer of 1989, continuing with the occasional foray into 1990 too. The so-called 'Acid House craze', in which very large numbers of people would congregate for parties in fields or in warehouses, led to media scares about the consumption of drugs, particularly psychedelics, which have been the subject of a revival along with associated forms of youth culture. The rise of Ecstasy and the reprise of LSD were not linked to crime in the same way as for example heroin (users said to commit crime to pay for their habit) and crack cocaine (users said to become violent, dealers said to be violent) have been. The dangerousness of psychedelics has been presented rather differently and includes the threat to the 'nation's youth' and profiteering by dealers in this new and lucrative market (Morton 1989: 2,120–1). Along with these have gone the problems of having unlicensed or unregulated parties (fire and other health and safety hazards) and the issue of 'traffic convoys' as large numbers of people have created traffic congestion. (Why this should be different from any other cause of congestion is unclear, especially as most of this happened late at night and at weekends when the roads should be relatively freer.)

A number of raids at parties led to hauls of quantities of psychedelic drugs, in turn fuelling the argument that behind it all were organised criminals supplying drugs to young people. A 'Regional pay party unit' was established to coordinate intelligence about the occurrence of Acid House parties around the M25 area and the Home Counties (Sapsted 1989: 2). Nor did this become a phenomenon confined to the south-east only, as in 1990 the

West Yorkshire police arrested over eight hundred people in a raid on a party near Leeds (Wainwright 1990: 1). Meanwhile, in 1989 one Member of Parliament had called for asset confiscation (to be described in Chapter 10) to be extended to the profits of party organisers (*Police Review* 1989b: 2,166). In July 1990 new legislation came into force which provided for fines of up to £20,000 and imprisonment for up to six months or both for the organisers of such parties (Home Office 1990c). In August 1990 an amendment to the Criminal Justice Act 1988 gave courts the power to confiscate the profits, where they exceed £10,000, of people convicted of offences against the new Act (Home Office 1990d). Here yet again, drugs legislation is seen to be the precursor for wider developments in the legal system. On the penalties side, one individual received a sentence of ten years for conspiracy to manage premises where he knew drugs would be supplied (*Police Review* 1989c: 2,314).

One example of such an exercise, which the media were invited to observe, is described by Kirby (1989c). An operation by the Number 3 Area Territorial Support Group was planned against a party underneath a railway arch in Camberwell in south London.

> [The officers] donned bullet and knife-proof body armour, flameproof overalls and visored steel helmets. . . . Then came the real instruments of battle, the siege equipment – a thermic lance, hydraulic ram, angle grinder and a sledgehammer. . . . There are 150 officers in the convoy – one for each partygoer. . . . Chief Insp[ector] Brian Younger tells Thames Television why the drink, drugs and undoubted fire risk make it important to crack down on such parties.
>
> (Kirby 1989c: 5)

Twenty-six people were arrested, eight of whom were later charged with drugs offences while another five were bailed awaiting the results of laboratory analysis (*ibid.*).

The Acid House raids are concerned with public disorder (even if it does arise after the police have intervened) and with the rather unusual attempt to intervene in drug consumption *at the point of use*. Thus they could be said to be having the dual effect of seeking to reduce the distribution of drugs and to curtail their consumption. In having both aims, they could be seen to go beyond any of the simple supply/demand reduction approaches more commonly to be found.

There have been several criticisms of this sort of raid. The *Guardian* (editorial, 1989b: 18) commented that

> The biggest danger of the parties, however, is the hype about their drug-pushing purpose. . . . The idea that the big drug barons are behind such events is absurd. The insidious barons are far too discreet to get involved in such brash, risky effusions. . . . The parties provide the police with the tempting illusion of drug action . . . the . . . biggest danger is that they will become a diversion from serious anti-drugs operations.

But, as we ask without any intended irony throughout this book, what is a serious anti-drugs operation? It is by no means clear that all down-market strategies are by definition not 'serious'. Each may have merits and demerits. Let us turn now to street sweeps.

Sweeps

Eck (1989b) describes sweeps as one of the methods which can be used by the police in targeting mid- to low-level dealers, including street dealers. A very overt method, this entails the police 'sweeping' blocks of the city which have become synonymous with drug dealing. Who gets 'swept up' is essentially unselective – 'everything that moves on two feet, and some on four, is arrested' (quoted in Eck 1989b: 8). Sweeping then is designed to disrupt localised markets simply by increasing the difficulty for sellers and buyers to make the deal.

> Sweeps produce a large number of arrests but the . . . evidence suggests that this strategy fails as often as it succeeds . . . successes are often fleeting. The costs of maintaining these operations can be quite high . . . [and] experimental evidence suggests that local residents do not notice any positive effects, and their fears of crime remain unchanged.
>
> (Eck 1989b: 9).

A more selective sweep is what Manning (1980) calls 'head-hunting', which involves cruising known drug-dealing areas and using an informant to point out suspected dealers, thought to have drugs on their person and then arresting the dealer.

A case study of disruptive policing involving the use of sweeps was Operation Pressure Point (OPP) on the Lower East Side of

New York City. In this area the trade had become sufficiently open for descriptions such as 'drugs supermarket' and 'the most open heroin market in the nation' (Zimmer 1987: 1). A combination of reasons made the area attractive to drug users and a difficult area to police. As the drug trade expanded it passed beyond the capacity of the local police and the assignment of Special Narcotic Enforcement Units was described as 'too little, too late' (Zimmer 1987: 3). Media and political interests focused attention on the area and in 1984 Operation Pressure Point was launched as a response. Primarily a uniformed police operation it entailed police foot patrols sweeping the streets, dispersing crowds, issuing parking tickets, and searching and arresting people. In addition operations were carried out on public housing projects, mounted police rode through the area, police dogs were used to search out empty and abandoned buildings, and hidden surveillance and 'buy and bust' operations were carried out by the organised Crime Control Bureau while helicopters hovered above watching for any attacks on the police (*ibid.*: 4–5). In addition courts handed out harsher penalties.

> Even when unable to make arrests, OPP forces tried to discourage involvement in the drug trade by acting as what Sagarin and McNamara (1972) call a 'judical punitive body'. This is a euphemism for harassing suspicious people in 'known drug areas' by stopping them, questioning them, perhaps searching them and telling them to 'move on'. From the police perspective, the advantage of this type of intervention is that it does not take officers off the street. The cost to the suspect is substantially less than with an arrest but a greater number of interventions per officer becomes possible.
>
> (Zimmer 1987: 6)

By increasing the risk of arrest for buyers and sellers, OPP led to changes in the pattern of trade. Buyers responded by spending less time on the streets and sellers varied the place and time of their sales, dealt in larger quantities and employed more helpers: 'steerers' notified buyers where and when sales would take place, 'lookouts' sent out warning signals when the police appeared (*ibid.*: 6–7). In other words, sweeps tend to apply pressure against those street dealers that we described in Chapter 4 above as 'irregulars', and leaves the door open to more organised 'retail specialists'. Such a development has been described as happening in areas of south London which have been subjected to this kind of policing (1989 interview with senior 'crack squad' officer).

For Zimmer, however, OPP has been a successful operation for the NY police because it has meant reduced drug dealing in the area, a change in the way in which dealing takes place (less overt), a displacement of some drug operations to other areas and a decrease in drug-related acquisitive crime. Zimmer also notes that the operation was more successful because the area was already undergoing gentrification and that a similar police operation in Harlem had little impact (*ibid.*: 17), and that 'early success occurred primarily because the drug traffic had become so blatant; now that buyers and sellers have had time to adjust to the police presence, law enforcement has become more difficult' (*ibid.*: 15). Sustained police pressure was required, without which the trade would rapidly re-emerge. More recently, street selling in New York City has been targeted by the Tactical Narcotics Team (or TNT) using saturation techniques (Marriott 1989).

Sweeps create high public expectations for the police, because other areas also want similar operations to improve their areas, without diminishing the resources and achievements of the operation which raised those expectations in the first place.

Another case of sweeping – this time in relation to organised gangs involved in drug dealing – is the work of the Los Angeles Police Department (LAPD). In 1988 the LAPD's Gang Related Active Trafficker Suppression (GRATS) programme carried out raids of 'drug neighborhoods' by squads of between 200 and 300 police (Davis 1988: 38–40). GRATS was succeeded by Operation Hammer, the 'thousand-cop blitzkriegs' (*ibid.*: 40). One thousand police officers were used to sweep the area. Over one thousand people were arrested, many for petty offences; others who were arrested but not charged had their name added to a roster for future surveillance (*ibid.*: 37). Unsurprisingly, the American Civil Liberties Union complained of extensive infringement of civil rights under Operation Hammer.

A further measure employed by the LAPD has been to declare some neighbourhoods as 'drug enforcement areas'. This entails blocking off streets with the intention of allowing only residents and their guests in. Although some success has been claimed, the police also say that the effect of this 'Neighborhood Rescue Operation' is that dealers have simply set up business in neighbouring areas. But, 'In the week after the barricades went up in one area, police arrested 40 drug buyers just four blocks away in a two-day undercover sweep' (Thompson 1989: 8). An LAPD officer said, 'It's like pushing an air bubble around inside an air mattress – it changes location, but it doesn't go away' (*ibid*.: 8). Here, once again, is the simple displacement effect of enforcement action in a particular area.

Street policing in Notting Hill

We turn now to the case of Notting Hill in west London as an example of police action in targeting a retail drug market. This example is particularly instructive in that it demonstrates that policing strategies are not always chosen and implemented by senior officers in a simple way. There are always constraints, some of which are internal to the police, and some external. Strategies evolve over time, changing as each new wave of personnel tries to overcome problems experienced with preceding strategies.

So, as with all police strategies in a particular place over time, it would be wrong to trace out a *consistent* police policy in Notting Hill. The question of what has been defined as the problem to be policed and the appropriate policing policy and strategy to respond to that problem is inevitably a process, and one which is heavily determined by the structural constraints within which the police operate, local pressures (pulling in different directions) and the particular social/historical context in which the police have been operating. Indeed the two examples from the 1980s which we shall go on to describe are two contrasting approaches to the policing of the area and to the locales of drug dealing.

Notting Hill is an area with a rich history, for many associated with the 1958 'race riots' and the annual carnival, both of which are part of the collective memory and struggles between black people and the police in the area (see for example Fryer 1984: 378–80 and 391–3). A focal point of those struggles has been the All Saints Road, characterised by the then Metropolitan Police Commissioner Sir Kenneth Newman as one of the 'symbolic locations' for policing in London. The association of All Saints Road with crime and drugs has been a touchstone of the police response to the road over a number of years. It has become an area where there have been open challenges to the police and in particular to police attempts to make arrests. To the fore have been the sustained allegations about police harassment of black people and the alleged association of black people with drugs, first with cannabis but, more damagingly in the 1980s, with cocaine and crack as well.

With regard to police activity in response to the perceptions of the street drug market in the All Saints Road, we shall look at two periods in the 1980s. Prominent during both periods have been questions about the style of policing and the relationship between the police and some local organisations.

Stage 1: the 'Black Watch' and 'fit-ups'

We begin with an account of the period 1982–5. The public disorders of 1981 had led to talk of 'sensitive' policing in racially mixed areas such as Notting Hill. This approach is exemplified in the 1982–4 period during which the Notting Hill police division was under the control of Chief Superintendent Whitfield. According to Keith (1986) Whitfield's policy was informed by the need to remove the 'symbolism' of All Saints Road, thereby demonstrating that the police were in control, since the road could be shown to be policed in the same way as any other part of London. To this end, Keith describes four measures taken by Whitfield to change the style of policing. First, he prevented cars from patrolling the road and ordered that cars from other divisions should not engage in 'hot pursuit' through the road. Keith (1986) comments that 'This was not popular with either junior officers or several skeptical superiors at Scotland Yard'.

Second, Whitfield's plan was to stop the mass police raids which frequently characterised police activity in the road and in particular against the Mangrove restaurant, which was viewed by local officers as a site for drug dealing. In their place came the use of more technological targeting and surveillance operations on the road. Third, Whitfield set up informal police–community liaison meetings, which included special one-off meetings about All Saints Road. Finally, and perhaps most significantly, from the end of the 1982 Carnival, Whitfield established a special patrol of twenty-four officers from Notting Hill who were detailed to 'recover' All Saints Road as an area of police control. Six officers would always be stationed in the road, twenty-four hours a day. According to Keith, despite local opposition this operation was moderately successful in reducing the number of people who 'frequented' the road.

Junior officers in the division were strongly critical of Whitfield's approach and the restrictions on their discretion to act. The All Saints Road patrol became increasingly detached from the rest of the Notting Hill division and somewhere around 1984 (at least some of) the patrol are reputed to have formed themselves into the notorious 'Black Watch', and are said to have taken the law into their hands acting as a vigilante group, subverting official policy by harassing black people and allegedly planting drugs on them (Keith 1986; Graef 1990: 27). Such activities did little to prevent drug trafficking, since

> In 1985 the Resident's Association of the newly refurbished St. Luke's Mews threatened to sue the police for their failure to enforce the law in the area (particularly drug trafficking).
>
> (Keith 1986)

The consequences of the years of the 'Black Watch' were a series of very public embarrassments for the Metropolitan Police, as three successful claims for damages followed from the wrongful arrest and malicious prosecution of three black men for alleged drug offences. In 1984 Rupert Taylor, a teetotal lay preacher, was wrongly arrested and prosecuted for possession of cannabis. Taylor took out in a civil case and in December 1989 he was awarded the record sum of £100,000 against the Metropolitan Police in damages for false imprisonment, malicious prosecution and exemplary damages (the amount was later reduced to £65,000). In July 1985 Vincent Lee was arrested for possession of five bags of cannabis. Lee was acquitted the next year and claimed that police officers had hit him over the head with a truncheon and planted the drugs on him. In November 1989 Lee was awarded £3,500 in damages by the High Court for assault, false imprisonment and malicious prosecution. In April 1985 Hughie Wilson, a trainee accountant, was arrested during raids on the Mangrove and alleged to have thrown cannabis on the floor. During a scuffle with the police Wilson injured his ribs and was severely bruised. He was charged with the possession of cannabis with intent to supply and with assault with intent to resist arrest but acquitted at Knightsbridge Crown Court in 1986. In March 1990 Wilson received £20,000 in damages in an out-of-court settlement with the Metropolitan Police for false arrest, unlawful imprisonment and malicious prosecution. Subsequently Notting Hill police became the subject of an inquiry by the Hertfordshire police and the Police Complaints Authority

(Kirby 1989b: 5; Graef 1990: 27; *IRR: Police–Media Research Project* 1990: 2; see also Levin 1990a: 14: Levin 1990b: 12).

Thus, the early 1980s illustrate a period in which the resistance of the lower ranks undermined more senior officers' attempts to carry out drug enforcement 'sensitively'.

Stage 2: Operation Trident

We now turn to the period from 1987 onwards, when Notting Hill was under the direction of Chief Superintendent Pearman. When Pearman came to Notting Hill the police perception of the All Saints Road and of the problem to be dealt with was clear to him and to other officers in his command.

> In 1987 when I first came here, the problem in the All Saints Road particularly was that you would have open street dealing going on almost in front of police officers, because literally hundreds of young blacks would congregate in streets off the All Saints Road and if police officers attempted to do anything there would be a public disorder situation on a daily basis.
>
> (Notting Hill police officer 1)

Pearman's view of the 'open to all comers' local drug market was that

> The drug culture encourages crime. People steal goods and cash to exchange for drugs. Back in March of '87, all crime problems focussed on the All Saints Road, yet the majority of arrests came from other parts of the country – even Europe. There were up to a thousand people there in clubs and bars – it was impossible to police. We had no access, no information.
>
> (Pearman in *The Hill*, 1989: 7)

Similarly, another Notting Hill officer said

> Bear in mind that it wasn't a residential market, it was people – okay some people were local – but by and large it was people from outside the area who came to buy . . . because it had a name, it had a reputation that if you want to buy drugs in London go to Notting Hill, go to All Saints Road.
>
> (Notting Hill officer 2)

In contrast with these accounts a local solicitor we interviewed saw the policing of the road rather differently: 'There is an observable

policy of shutting down activities around the All Saints Road area
. . . it's high-profile policing, there are vans racing up and down
the road'.

In response to the street drug market, Pearman launched
Operation Trident, an extensive surveillance operation aimed
at suspected drug dealers, in June 1987. A Notting Hill officer
described the operation and located it within the 'corporate
approach' that Pearman espoused.

Operation Trident was implemented in June 1987 and that was
basically an observation exercise where they used four covert
observation posts, and watched the street dealing and logged
all the movements and the people that bought the drugs were
in the main arrested, and then by doing that we built up a
dossier on each of the dealers and at the end of June we
went out and arrested them. We arrested seventeen dealers
at that time and convicted eleven of them and I think that in
that case there were 144 buyers of drugs who were arrested
during that observation as well. Following that operation there
was quite a large influx of uniformed police into the area and
it was then really that things started to alter – there were a lot
of other things that happened in the area, a lot of renovation
work and things like that were done by the Task Force. Basically
they were moving a lot of these doorways out to stop people
having these little hidey-holes where they could deal drugs and
things like that – so it was really a multi-agency approach sort
of concept, it wasn't just the police out to try and change
things, there was a lot of help from the community generally.
And then at that time the police tried to get more involved
in the community . . . because I think that up to that time
most police officers at this station considered that most of the
community in that area were quite hostile to us, it wasn't in
fact until we got there and spoke to people that you realise
that 95 per cent of people were very much on our side and
have probably been waiting for years for us to do this sort of
thing.

(Notting Hill officer 1)

Here – as in the case of raids – local public support is seen
as an important source of legitimation for police actions. Law
enforcement in such circumstances is commended by Moore and
Kleiman (1989) in their discussion of 'neighborhood crackdowns'.

> The police might decide to leverage their resources by cracking down on drug offenses in those neighborhoods that are willing to join the police in resisting drug use. . . . Police resources would be attracted to those areas precisely because there is some prospect that the impact of police crackdown would be prolonged and widened by determined citizens.
>
> (Moore and Kleiman 1989: 9)

In the case of Notting Hill it remains a moot point whether the police 'lead' or 'follow' the community, apart from the far more intractable issue of who 'the community' to be consulted and considered actually are.

Following Operation Trident, the police suspected that trafficking might have been driven off the street and displaced into buildings. Operation Buccaneer 2 in August 1989 involved about eighty police officers – in nine vans and an unmarked lorry – raiding two premises in the area. Seventeen people were arrested, but only one was charged with drug dealing. Three others were charged with possession but the remainder were either charged with public order offences or released without charge (McDermott 1989: 7).

Stage 3: Operation Mint

Operation Mint, which took place between November and December 1989, was the last major drugs operation in Pearman's time at Notting Hill (his successor took over in January 1990) and a smaller-scale version of Operation Trident, which was seen by some local officers as the starting point for police activity in the latter period of the 1980s.

> So that was where it all started to turn round and I think the operations we're doing now follow on from it.
>
> (Notting Hill officer 1)
>
> Yes that did turn it around and the number of people in the street gradually reduced . . . it became less of a symbolic location if you like for people to congregate. . . . I mean because there's undoubtedly a cultural aspect to it as well, where people met socially as well as the drug problem, so we'd ran [a number of] sort of small operations following Trident.
>
> (Notting Hill officer 2)

Operation Mint was described by these Notting Hill officers as 'basically centred around the All Saints Road'. This account is based on their account as the officers primarily responsible for the management of that operation.

Around about October last year [1989] various individuals began to look at the street and come to me and say 'I think so and so's drug dealing', there were different outfits in the police station as well as outside the police station saying it was time we did something, so I decided that it was time we needed to get the interested parties together. . . . Instead of having splintered operations we decided that we would go and do a similar operation to Trident and we obtained a couple of covert locations [at the end of] last year. That was an interesting exercise in itself because up to that point you have individual perceptions of how bad the problem is or where the problem is focused upon . . . different premises are popped up as being the centre. But we ran a pilot observation just to find out what the problem was – for about a week – and we did nothing with the information we gathered other than use it as pure intelligence.

We brought that back here and looked at it and we decided that the way forward was to run an OP [observation post] for three weeks, Monday to Friday, for most of the day, late morning till midnight. During that time we recorded 123 deals of which sixty-four people were followed away from the street and arrested for possession. Now that was for cannabis and cocaine and crack, there were about a dozen deals or so of crack and there might have been the odd one of heroin, but heroin was conspicuous by its absence, so in the main we were dealing with cocaine and any derivatives of it and cannabis. The 123 deals were all dealt by sixteen different individuals, so although we had a slightly lesser number of total deals we were fairly close to the same number of dealers as Operation Trident, which was a very large police operation.

(Notting Hill officer 1)

The case built up by Operation Mint relied heavily on the detailed observation logs filled out by officers on surveillance. Photographs of deals taking place were not possible because the production of the photographs in court would reveal the observation site. This can be a common problem in surveillance operations, although in other cases the police have used video film and produced it as evidence. The logs included details about physical exchanges and the clothes that alleged dealers were wearing. Subsequently a coordinated police 'swoop' operation led to the arrest of most of the sixteen individuals, with the remainder being arrested afterwards.

> We set a particular morning when we would arrest everyone early in the morning at their home address. Now bear in mind that this was a different sort of drugs raid – we had warrants for all sixteen people. We weren't actually going looking for drugs, we were actually going to arrest sixteen people that we already had a prima facie case against for dealing in dangerous drugs. Now . . . we recovered fairly reasonable sums of money from these dealers' addresses. We also got the bonus of extra drugs on some of them.
>
> (Notting Hill officer 1)

At their houses the police photographed their clothes which matched the descriptions on the logs, to be produced as evidence in court. At the time of writing, thirteen out of the sixteen people had been remanded in custody for up to six months in 1990. For the police, a substantial gain of the operation that, regardless of eventual outcomes of court cases, the street was 'cleared' for six months whilst the accused were held on remand.[17]

> One of the most significant parts of the operation . . . [is that] apart from any other effects, the operation has actually removed sixteen dealers from the All Saints Road from December to May . . . so whatever the eventual outcome may be, we've achieved our objective because we can see a marked difference in the level of drug activity between December to May 1990 from December to May 1989. We've got six months of . . . it really is reduced – it was only in April that we found any sort of significant activity.
>
> (Notting Hill officer 1)

This form of preventive custody is indeed worthy of note. There is nothing improper in it in the eyes of British law, the prosecution merely having to convince a court that remand while awaiting trial is justified in the light of the available evidence. How the magistrates may in such circumstances weigh the case for and against remand is another matter.

One particularly interesting and unreported aspect of Operation Mint (and possibly other such operations elsewhere in Britain) is that, for the two days prior to arresting the alleged traffickers, the police followed drug purchasers out of the area and quietly arrested them. It is to be expected that, returning to their areas of residence, these purchasers told their acquaintances that Notting Hill was 'bad news'. Here then is one form of law enforcement involvement in demand reduction. It is this part of a local story which takes us to the wider framework of international drug control policy.

TARGETING THE PURCHASER

The basis of so-called demand reduction policies is that if there were no potential buyers then there would be no market for sellers to offer their wares to. While demand reduction is usually conceived of as being something to do with education and, sometimes, treatment, it might appear to have little to do with law enforcement per se. However, the targeting of drug purchasers – most explicitly in the notion of their 'moral responsibility' for patronising the drug trade – does represent a form of demand reduction in action.

One of the main points of former US 'Drug Czar' William Bennett's drug control strategy (Office of National Drug Control Policy 1989; Lichfield 1989: 6) is that drug users should be made accountable for their role in maintaining the drug trade.[18] For Bennett, the answer in the war on drugs is the reconstitution of social, political and moral authority. Drug offenders must believe in the inevitability of punishment: 'As long as they don't, the deterrent effect of incarceration will be neutralized' (Bennett 1989: 5). And,

> This holds true, perhaps even more true, for the non-addicted user, the so-called 'casual user.' Casual use is not just a matter of personal preference. It has costs – wide, horrible social costs. The suburban man who drives his BMW downtown to buy cocaine is killing himself, of course. But he is killing the city at the same time. And his 'casual' use is best deterred not by empty threats of long, hard punishment, but by *certain* punishment. Compel him, as authorities are doing in Phoenix, to pay a steep fine and spend a weekend in jail. Seize his BMW right after he has bought some dope, and when he is convicted, take the car away from him for good. That is what they do in Philadelphia.
>
> (*ibid.*: 5)

Bennett may speak of certain rather than severe punishment, but in this gung-ho climate, severity never seems very far away. For example, for first-time offenders 'boot camp' is proposed, 'because it is so grueling and unpleasant' (*ibid.*).

This consumer-led, demand-oriented conceptualisation of the drug problem has significant consequences. It establishes a notion of moral culpability, justifying the stringent measures to be employed in work place drug testing, in which employee cooperation becomes a criterion for career advancement (Hecker and Kaplan 1989). In the US, drug testing is being suggested in educational institutions and in the criminal justice system as a precondition for receiving federal funds, and states could be given the power to revoke drivers' licences for those failing a test.[19] Court guidelines have been issued which give federal and state courts the discretion to deny eligibility to a wide range of federal benefits to individuals convicted of possession offences (*Alcoholism and Drug Abuse Week* 1990: 7). For Bennett, 'This law reflects a proper assumption, in my view, that persons found guilty of drug crimes should, at the very least, forfeit their claims to taxpayer-conferred status and non-essential economic benefits' (*ibid.*). The constitutionality of some of these measures and the 'drugs exception' to the US constitution have been queried (Wisotsky 1987).

A study by Reuter *et al.* (1990) suggests that if this strategy is to be pursued, then police activity against *purchasers* may be more effective in cutting demand than a general anti-user sweep envisaged by the Bennett plan, or a continuation of the current anti-trafficker focus.

> If we accept that street dealers' high earnings are only explainable by the existence of a large middle-class market (as our data suggest), then exploring the desirability of sanctions against those who patronize the street markets is of considerable interest.
>
> (Reuter *et al.* 1990: 108)

This then is an alternative to the 'general user sanctions' anticipated by the Bennett plan. The suggestion is that police activities could be more effectively targeted at 'affluent' buyers who use street markets because they are an anonymous trading place. Such buyers are more likely to feel the deterrent effect (presumably because of their otherwise 'respectable' backgrounds) of having criminal records and receiving financial penalties or being imprisoned. If this worked and affluent buyers stop using street markets, this in turn would make those markets less profitable for sellers (Reuter *et al.* 1990: 108; Denniston 1990a).

Inconvenience policing

The idea of hitting the drug trade by making things more difficult for purchasers is not new. A similar approach was previously advocated by Moore (1977: 239–47), especially in relation to novice heroin users who are

> quite vulnerable to changes, even small ones, in the availability of heroin . . . a person who has not yet become a heavy user will not conduct an intensive search for a supply. Some studies have suggested that a 'dabbler' may use heroin if it is immediately available, but will not use it if it requires two, three, or four hours of searching. Extending the search time for novices may discourage or reduce the frequency of their use of heroin.
>
> (Wilson 1985: 214)

Under these conditions, intensified policing could lead dealers to abandon their traditional sites of supply or make them more cautious about dealing to unfamiliar buyers (on the grounds that the new buyers may be undercover police working to a 'buy bust' policy). In either case the effect of police activity is to make life considerably more difficult for dealers and in particular for casual or novice buyers.

> Heroin customers can be thought of as a 'queue' with the heaviest users at the head of the line and the casual ones at the end; how far down the queue the dealer will do business depends on the perceived level of risk associated with each additional customer, and that in turn depends on how strongly 'the heat is on'.
>
> (Wilson 1985: 214)

The idea of 'inconvenience policing' then is to deter the casual buyer by increasing the 'search time' which it will take her/him to find heroin. One important base for this strategy is the realisation that the effects of law enforcement may drive up the street price of a drug over the long term, but that this is not the only way in which enforcement can impact on the drug market. As Wilson (1985: 214) concludes – 'in the short term, anti-dealer law enforcement probably affects access (finding a "connection") more than price.'

Inconvenience policing, like any other approach, has its costs. As Hughes *et al.* (1971: 43) found

[Dealing] locations are frequently under police surveillance, [so] the addict cannot walk up to a dealer, pass him money, and walk away. Therefore copping communities tend to develop a rather complex organization to protect their membership from constant police pressure. In this way they resemble delinquent gangs and other criminal organizations.

Again, we see one of the ways in which law enforcement shapes the market, here pushing low-level dealing into the relatively organised form of the 'retail specialist'.

TARGETING THE USER

Within the American debate and its European echoes it is possible to distinguish a range of positions regarding action against drug users/purchasers.

The 'toughest' stand is being articulated by Judge Robert Bonner, the new administrator of the DEA who advocates incarceration – even for possession of small amounts for personal use – on the grounds that it would get those people off drugs, even if temporarily. In anticipation of the obvious counter-argument about the availability of drugs in prisons, Bonner adds that extra measures should be used to prevent drug smuggling into prisons (*Drug Enforcement Report* 1990b: 6). By contrast, the most refined version of this targeting the drug purchaser approach is Reuter *et al.*'s (1990) argument that the effect of targeting affluent purchasers is likely to prove to be the most effective means of changing the nature of street markets. In between these two positions lies an emerging middle ground of opinion, which sees little merit in packing out already overcrowded prisons with drug users and does not wish to restrict control to the point of purchase. This middle ground foresees an alliance between the criminal justice system and the health and welfare agencies, with the aim of pushing drug users into treatment.

Sentenced to treatment

Wilson (1985), Pearson (1989) and Gilman and Pearson (1991) among others have proposed that street enforcement could be based on the intention of arresting users and diverting them into treatment programmes.

One can imagine a variety of law-enforcement strategies that could have a powerful effect on the number of addicts on the street, and thus on the number of street crimes that they might commit and other harm that they might do to others and themselves. One could arrest every known addict and send him to a 'heroin quarantine center' with . . . intensive care programs. Or one could arrest every known addict and send him back onto the street under a 'pledge' system requiring him to submit to frequent urine tests which, if omitted or failed, would then lead to confinement in either center or jail.

(Wilson 1985: 211)

Similarly Gilman and Pearson (1991) have derided the 'myth of voluntarism' in explaining how and why people use drug advice services, and described ways in which law enforcement activity can persuade drug users to take 'early retirement' from their drug careers. Such measures can then be justified on law enforcement or health and welfare criteria, or both. For Johnson, 'Compulsory treatment is probably the most effective way to control the largest number of criminally active heroin users . . . people tend to reduce their criminality substantially while in treatment but not necessarily after release from prison or after treatment' (Johnson 1989: 12).

This 'sentenced to treatment' approach has already been operating in various parts of the US for a number of years, but is still at the 'drawing board' stage in Britain. Government proposals in Green and White Papers have suggested that instead of custodial sentences addicts could be diverted into treatment programmes linked to some form of conditional probation order (Home Office 1990a). It seems that we are embarking on a new approach in which, for at least some drug users, treatment and sentencing are to be co-joined.

CONCLUSION

As Chapters 5, 6 and 7 have shown, the development of anti-trafficking enforcement has been something of a pillar-to-post affair. The loudly announced war on 'big traffickers' is still being waged, though more in a spirit of dogged determination than optimism. The various middle-market strategies have yet to be fully tried out in either the United States or Britain, we think. Finally, the renewed interest in retail level action from street sweeps, through more selective action against retail traffickers, purchasers and consumers, has yet to be seriously appraised.

Now there are those who would blithely say that what is needed is more of *all* of these activities – underpinned by more money, more equipment, more personnel, more operations, more publicity. This is what Moore and Kleiman (1989: 6) call *expressive* law enforcement.

> This . . . takes all the activities in which the [police] department is engaged and increases them by a factor of two or three. If a city's drug problem is getting worse, the response is simply to increase the resources devoted to the problem.

For Moore and Kleiman this appeals on various grounds. It is a common-sense approach that is widely understood. It is a strategy which fits well with the interests of everybody working in drug enforcement. It may lead to the detention and eventual imprisonment of a large number of drug traffickers. Finally, it shores up general social hostility to drugs.

> [But] this strategy also has weaknesses. First it does not admit that police resources, even when multiplied, may not control the problem. It ignores . . . the rest of the [criminal justice] system; disregards the scale and resilience of the drug markets; and fails to establish any benchmarks for success other than the promise of a valiant effort to increase arrests.
>
> (*ibid.*: 6)

Today, although there are signs that the 'more of everything' approach still holds much appeal, it has run up against questions about whether or not it delivers the goods as promised and about the resource implications. In other words, people are beginning to ask that most unwelcome question, about cost-effectiveness.

In the third part of this book we examine some of the key issues for drug enforcement activity in the 1990s, including some activities, such as informant handling, drugs intelligence and imprisonment of drug traffickers, which seem relatively insensitive to resource constraints.

Part III

Key issues in drug enforcement

Chapter 8

Informants and stings
Tradition and innovation in plainclothes work

Part III focuses on three important issues in drug enforcement. In this chapter we look at detectives who, traditionally, have been regarded as the 'elite' of the police. The relations between detectives and their informants remain full of promise and danger. Chapter 9 describes the ascendancy of a rising elite – intelligence officers. Drugs intelligence constitutes the means whereby detective work is becoming directed from the centre. Finally, in Chapter 10 we examine penalties.

In discussing any profession, it is important to recognise that formal, structural aspects are at best half the story of any organisation: the informal aspects, sometimes referred to as 'occupational culture' (see Reiner 1985; Holdaway 1989) are just as important. Indeed, there may be grounds for saying that, the more formalised and hierarchical an organisation appears in formal terms, the more important informal understandings, linkages and procedures are in making it work. This is an important issue in detective work, particularly in relation to informant handling and covert operations. On the one hand there are acceptably creative interpretations of formal rules and regulations. On the other there are ways of working that come to be defined as unacceptable because either they result in successful legal challenges by defence lawyers in court, or they cause difficulties for other enforcement officers and operations, or they may become indistinguishable from corruption. The line between creativity and corruption can be a narrow one.

Detective work is where officers are seen as exhibiting the skills and proficiency which demarcate the exciting and sometimes dangerous aspect of the job, from the routine and the mundane reality of everyday work (Skolnick 1966; Reiner 1985). In this chapter we examine the key to success in detective work: the relationship with informants. The principal skill required by the officer is the ability to develop, maintain and act upon information that can be gleaned from informants. Informants, as we describe below, come in different types and with varying motives. Partly because of the complexity of this motivation, informant handling is considered one of the most important skills of a detective, and an area in which the officer must be thoroughly professional in order to avoid 'coming unstuck'.

The utility of informants often extends beyond the giving of information, and provides an important link into the types of undercover operations discussed in Chapter 6. There we described a 'buy bust' operation which involved an informant introducing an undercover officer to a prospective supplier of drugs. Below we look in more detail at the involvement of informants in buy operations, one of the most sensitive aspects of informant handling.

This chapter closes with an examination of a method that is officially denied to exist in Britain – 'sell operations' – some of which involve informants. A sell operation can be a simple 'sell bust', in which the police make an immediate arrest, or it can be part of a longer-term intelligence-gathering operation, aiming to ensnare a wider number of traffickers. Some other countries, notably the United States, have legitimised such operations and one of the questions for the 1990s is whether there will be pressure for similar powers to be granted here. Because of the extreme sensitivity of the issue, our discussion of it is informed partly by unattributable briefings, elaborated by surmise. However unsatisfactory such a state of affairs may be, we believe that any way into a more open discussion of this area is justified.

INFORMANTS AND THEIR HANDLERS

The importance of informants

[An informant is] any non-law enforcement person who, by reason of his familiarity or close association with criminals, supplies regular or constant information about criminal activities to a police officer.

(Drug Enforcement Administration 1982: 55)

The policing of drugs is distinguished by the absence of a complaining victim, which requires a reactive response from the police. Drugs are therefore part of that area usually called victimless or consensual crimes. The uniqueness of drug law enforcement work is precisely the necessity for proactive policing, in which the image of the 'narc' is constructed. As Skolnick says,

> Crimes without citizen complaints result in a structure demanding independent action on the policeman's part, and therefore emphasize the craftsmanlike possibilities of policework.
>
> (Skolnick 1966: 138)

This situation requires the police to position themselves into a distinct relation with the drug market in order to obtain information about activities within the market. It means that cases have to be initiated and made by narcotics officers (Skolnick 1966; Wilson 1978; Manning 1980). The single most important way of making drug cases is the use and development of informants.

> Narcotics agents must create their own workload by inducing individuals to reveal information they would prefer to keep confidential. (Wilson 1978: 57)
>
> The most important source of cases are those he [the agent] constructs himself or develops in concert with or as a result of interaction with an informant.
>
> (Manning 1980: 140)

The importance of informants is widely acknowledged (for instances, see Pritchard and Laxton 1978; Fuqua 1978; Williams and Guess 1981; Drug Enforcement Administration 1982; US General Accounting Office 1984: Home Affairs Committee 1989b). For drug agents, policing would be virtually impossible without informants. For example, Moore describes the police following 'leads'

> [Police] forces following the strategy of prospective investigation will restrict their attention to very specific, very reliable leads. These are most likely to come from informants or undercover activities.
>
> (Moore 1977: 136–7)

In this situation the prime task for officers is to establish relations with informants. For Manning (1980) 'the recruitment, interrogation, working and protection of informants is a focal or key activity in narcotics work'. Similarly in his comparative study of FBI and DEA agents Wilson says that

> The critical skill of a narcotics agent is the ability to persuade a person involved in crime to supply information that is not ordinarily to his advantage to reveal or to engage in a transaction that is not his interest to consummate.
>
> (Wilson 1978: 47)

But, paradoxically, even though an officer's skill in developing informants is a crucial determinant of success, little or no effort has been invested in finding out what this skill is and how it might be taught to others. As Wilson notes

> Informant development is, for DEA agents, a skill as important as interviewing methods for FBI agents, yet there is little evidence that either organization attempts systematically to discover why some have the skill or to develop that skill in others.
>
> (Wilson 1978: 51)

A similar picture applies in Britain. On his first day with the drug squad, Pritchard was simply told to get on with it.

> Drugs squad is supposed to be specialised, but there's no instructor to tell you what to do. No-one wants to know me. 'Go on. Piss off and get me some information.' And that's that.
>
> (Pritchard and Laxton 1978: 21)

Judging by our discussions with detectives in drug squads throughout Britain, Pritchard's experience may well be representative of the past. But senior officers are increasingly aware that relations between informants and their detective 'handlers' are fraught with dangers, if not overseen and regulated. Some of these dangers will be touched upon in this chapter. However, it remains the case that the often highly individualised relationship between officer and informant constitutes a key part of the detective tradition.

> They [agents] have learned to see their possibilities for success as dependent on identifying, cultivating, working and maintaining their informants. They assume this is the most fruitful way of working, in large part because they have never done anything else, have received little or no formal training . . . and because it is part of the traditional lore of the units that informants are the sine qua non of narcotics work.
>
> (Manning 1980: 141)

Why do they do it? Amateurs and professionals

Never trust an informant.

(Fuqua 1978: 176)

For Grieve (1987), informers are of two types: the professional informer or the public spirited. This is a distinction which pervades the categorisation of information. For example, a Drug Enforcement Administration (DEA) categorisation system distinguishes Class I informants who have criminal connections or background, from Class II informants, who are members of the public who have seen something suspicious and report it (Wilson 1978: 62).

Public-spirited informers are not always regarded as welcome. Although they are certainly plentiful (as calls to telephone lines like Crimestoppers demonstrate), their reasons are likely to be varied, including malice and self-aggrandisement. Similar cynicism about amateur informants has been noted in the United States.

> FBI and DEA agents alike often complain (never publicly) about public-spirited citizens, many of whom are 'police buffs' . . . and who call frequently to recount useless information and baseless suspicions . . . the self-appointed 'informant' is usually greeted with weary dismay.
>
> (Wilson 1978: 65)

The 'police buffs' are the types whose motivation according to one drug squad officer is that 'I'd love to do your job'. Williams and Guess (1981: 238) add that such information is rarely of any value and the informant is often discounted. The important difference between the two types of informers is that the professional informer may be being paid by the police or working in exchange for some return, which may or may not be specified. In this case, as Manning says, the informant must stand in some formal relationship to the police officer and 'this relationship distinguishes "citizens" from "informants"' (Manning 1980: 141).

The inducement of money in motivating both amateur and professional informers appears straightforward enough. One opinion is that 'The number of people who would "sell their own mothers up the river" for a few dollars is amazing. There will always be those individuals who regard informing as a convenient way of making money' (Fuqua 1978: 173). Recent ventures, such as 'Crimestoppers' in Britain, play upon this appeal to both 'public-spirited' and 'professional' informants. Rewards for assisting the police are paid by the Community Action Trust (CAT).[20] In 1990 CAT announced an extension of its activities through 'Drug Command', described as 'a scheme for assisting the Police to solve drug related crimes'.[21] Practically this means that informants can expect larger rewards than they could ever get from police funds if their information leads to a major dealer. Speculation about figures suggests that maximum rewards could rise from £3,000 to £100,000 (*Guardian* editorial 1990a: 18). The head of the Metropolitan Police's Central Drugs Squad was unreserved in welcoming this. It 'could make a hell of a difference. I'm in favour of anything that can make more money available for informants' (*ibid.*).[22]

Nevertheless, even large financial inducements may be insufficient. Williams and Guess (1981) found that a sense of privacy and a feeling of 'not wanting to get involved' often act as disincentives to becoming informants.

Professional informers

Fuqua (1978: 173–5) warns officers that an informant's motives need to be carefully assessed. The range of motives could include money, fear of prosecution, revenge and the elimination of competition (see also Williams and Guess 1981). Officers need to be on their guard against the possibility that an informant may have been 'fed' to them by dealers who are gathering information about police operations in which the informant might participate, or that the informant forms part of a set-up designed to entrap an officer in some way (Fuqua 1978). Tip-offs received from informants are seldom altruistically motivated.

> Due to the special nature of drug investigations . . . many informants do not have the most laudable motives. Many desire to avoid punishment for past misconduct, to gain revenge, or to obtain money. Some are facing arrest and criminal charges. Consequently [we] must use extreme caution when handling and dealing with informants of questionable character.
>
> (Raezer 1987: 39)

Professional informants are important precisely because of their association with the drug market and/or other forms of criminal activity (Williams *et al.* 1979: 33). It is of course one of the paradoxes of informant-based policing that the more valuable the information that can be imparted by the informant the more likely it is that s/he has been or is involved in criminal activity in a significant way. As Williams and Guess (1981: 240) put it, 'In essence the informant needs to be "dirty" to be useful'.

For informants too there is a need to form a relationship with one or particular officers. For Frank, a professional police informer

> Motivation is an odd thing. I mean it's very difficult to form a relationship with the police because you're a criminal and I've had a certain amount of experience with the police and obviously there's been some cock-ups and nasty mess along the way, know what I mean. So it's very difficult to form any sort of relationship with a police officer unless you're lucky enough to be accepted. I mean if you've got a genuine desire to do good then this can make a great difference. If there's any bullshit then I can drop out – I *don't have* to help them.

Informants are obviously aware of their importance to the police. For example, officers may be reliant on the informants to provide a lead, but there could easily be ulterior reasons for giving that lead.

> He [the officer] can't know what's going on unless I tell him. And I might be telling him for all different reasons. You know [I might say] 'so and so is doing this', because they've upset me [the informant]. Then . . . the police . . . go and give them some aggravation.
>
> (Frank)

For Frank, as a minor dealer himself, there is also the knowledge that being an informer does not necessarily afford any protection against being under surveillance by the police – whether it is officers in the same squad as the informant's handler, or in another squad who stumble across the dealing activities of the informer and are unaware that he is an informer. Frank was unsure where he stood in these respects, expressing the hope that 'his' officer would, if he were able, tell the informant of the surveillance so that he would have the chance to abstain from risky activity at such times.

You know, if you're under observation then you're under observation. You'd like – you'd probably know – I hope you'd *have* to know [that you are under surveillance].

Where do professional informants come from?

A narc is only as good as his snitches.
(officer quoted by Manning and Redlinger 1978: 64)

Since the most useful informants are those with direct knowledge of drug markets through their own participation in it, most if not all drug arrestees can expect to be asked for information. It is in the period of questioning an arrested drug dealer that the officer has the opportunity to try to persuade the suspect to 'flip' into an informant (Wilson 1978: 73; Williams *et al*. 1979: 34). In Britain the usual terms are 'turn' or 'roll'.

The questioning session is almost always a one-sided affair, with the police officer having the authority and knowledge of the law while the arrested person will often lack both of those, as well as being in a vulnerable situation. One option available to the officer in this situation is to plea bargain informally with the person in custody.

Ninety-nine per cent of all our informants come from arrests and we . . . turn to those dealers to give us other details. . . . His Lord Chief Justice laid down . . . guidelines to other judges and basically what he says is that if they do the right thing, you won't have to bang them up for quite as long as you would have.

(drug squad officer)

What can a cooperative informant expect from the police by 'doing the right thing'? For a cooperative informant who is tried the police prepare three copies of a report known as the confidential text.[23] In the Metropolitan Police, one copy goes to New Scotland Yard and another to the Crown Prosecution Service. (This is a relatively new procedure and the police dislike doing this since they regard it as a security risk.) A third copy goes to the trial judge who may say something like 'I have read the reports on you' before passing sentence on an informant who has been prosecuted and found guilty.

Informants are most likely to be persuaded to 'turn' or 'flip' by being offered some exchange of mitigation or leniency. Wilson notes that, 'A major motive – most investigators believe *the* major motive – of an informant is to obtain leniency on a criminal charge in exchange for information about accomplices involved' (Wilson 1978: 65). In American parlance such informants are described as 'working off a beef', 'cooperating in exchange for having charges dropped or lessened, or milder sentences imposed, on criminal matters they faced' (*ibid.*: 65; see also Williams and Guess 1981: 239). In Wilson's study the majority of informants were 'working off a beef'. Similarly, Bakalar and Grinspoon (1984: 112) have noted that most often 'the key to drug law enforcement is the use of informers who cooperate to reduce their own sentences'. And Fuqua (1978: 174) adds that

> These are the individuals who become informants in an attempt to save their own skins. More often than not such an informant is a small-time operator who is facing a charge and who hopes either to get it dismissed or to get off with a suspended or light sentence in return for cooperation.[24]

Other informant motives described by Wilson (1978) included seeking money (the professional informer) and ideological reasons (in Wilson's study, anti-communist feelings) but these may prove to be transient motives. Wilson (1978: 66) found that agents believed that people 'working off a beef' are more likely to become long-term informants. They also have the added advantage of being the more economical, since the nature of the deal between them and the criminal justice system means that financial incentives are not usually required. Their dependence on the police is also said to make them more reliable than informants who may be paid more but are less vulnerable to police pressure (Williams *et al*. 1979: 35).

For the informer, the 'pay-off' may extend from receiving a reduced sentence to being allowed to continue operating under some degree of police supervision – minor dealing in exchange for regular information. In some cases, as we shall see in describing informant-related operations, an informant may do a great deal more than this and even become a participant in a police operation.

INFORMANTS AND OPERATIONS

According to Wilson (1978: 62) criminal informants can serve three functions for the police.

One is simply as a source of leads as to the behaviour of a suspect, the identity of a violator or the location of the loot. A second is to deceive other criminals by introducing them to undercover agents pretending to be criminals or by stimulating would-be offenders to commit a crime while being observed by agents. These are sometimes called 'participating informants'. A third is to testify in court against criminal accomplices; these are referred to as 'informant defendants'.

Informants' leads

Elaborating on Wilson's first category of informant, a drug squad officer described informant leads about addresses from which dealing occurs as of only limited value.

> The one that tells us Fred Bloggs at such and such an address is dealing. If you take a score from one to ten as to that information, I would put that down at about two or three. OK let's say the information is true, then you set up your observation point and we do this purely by leg work, by police work. 'Thanks for the information we will sort that out'. [So you] set up your observation point and sit and watch it. The factors that can assist you as to whether you are going to get a good hit or not are such things as, yes there has been three people at the door, they were there a short time. The balance of probabilities is that they were punters. So then let's go back tomorrow, yes we have got one punter who we recognise from the day before.

Having such a basis on which to believe that drugs are being supplied, there are two possible courses of action open to the police. The first is to raid the house, but that is an expensive course of action in resource terms. It would normally only be countenanced if there were strong indications – that is, evidence over and above the word of the informant – that significant quantities of drugs would be found. A second possibility is for an undercover officer to effect an introduction to the dealer and to solicit a sale. This too can be time consuming except in the case of incautious dealers. Furthermore, there are many circumstances in which a person who is trafficking will simply be unable to supply their new 'customer'.

> You go in there [the house] and they will say 'Yeah I am a dealer, sorry I didn't have any gear, the first punter arrived and I sent him away because I didn't have any gear'. Absolutely true.

Another option is to follow the buyer.

> We can say . . . we will let the punters go a mile away and pull them. I don't like doing that because what happens if he has got nothing on him, you have to let him go. He is straight round to a phone box, saying 'I have had a pull' and the gear goes down the toilet.

So the informant whose cooperation is limited to giving leads is considered by many officers to be 'useful [but also] very time consuming'. Many officers believe that such an informant is likely to be really useful only at the lowest levels of the market.

Participating informants

Grieve (1987: 453) defines a participating informant as one 'whose role goes beyond mere observation and reporting and whose activities are recorded and controlled by police so they may subsequently be professionally or legally assessed'. Such cooperation is highly valued by drug squad officers.

> [This type of informant] is the one I like. It is the participating informant . . . where it is very very strictly controlled. It is where I put on paper [report to senior officers] that I have an informant and I want him to participate in a very minor role in crime. They are the best informants in the world, because they can literally go into a dealer's address, come out and run their fingers through their hair and that is the signal [that] he is sitting there with a mountain of the stuff. Give him [the informant] half an hour to get away or maybe even arrest him as he is coming out. The important thing is . . . to protect him [the informant]. That is the best informant in the world and we have . . . used a number of those highly successfully. Tremendously successful.
>
> (drug squad officer)

An example of a case involving a participating informant case is Greg, whom we described in Chapter 4 as a retail specialist. After being arrested in possession of about six ounces of cocaine, Greg agreed to be a party to a police buy operation targeting Smith, a

London-based importer, and Paul, the 'runner' for Smith. Under instructions and surveillance by the police, Greg used his portable phone to call Paul and arrange to be supplied with eight ounces of cocaine. Paul said that he would call back within an hour to arrange the delivery point. However, the portable phone did not work again after this call was made, according to Greg because the police 'jammed' it to prevent further communication. The police used the first call to trace Paul and raided that address. Paul had himself become suspicious about Greg's jammed telephone line and had hidden the cocaine before the raid, but the police still found substantial quantities of cannabis and amphetamines at the house. A subsequent raid at Smith's house was too late and he was thought to have left the country.

On the subject of communications, another sort of participating informant is familiar to watchers of American cop movies. In a discussion about the use of electronic surveillance, Raezer (1987: 12) uses the term 'consensual informant' to describe a person wearing a 'wire' to record a conversation to be replayed as evidence in court. There is considerable debate in the US about the admissibility of evidence thus obtained and Supreme Court rulings delineate the area of 'privacy' protected. There is no constitutional right to privacy as such in Britain.

Taking out the competition

A danger in police–informant relations is that the informant who is also trafficking tries to use the police to eliminate competitors (Fuqua 1978: 174–5).

> The dealer [and informant] who is out on bail . . . thinks to himself, 'I have got a police officer who is handling me, what am I going to do, I am going to continue dealing, but I am going to be a little bit shrewder so that he [the officer] don't find out'. And it is like any other business, [the informant thinks] 'why don't I in order to get my little bit of a favour at court, take out my opposition'. Because all the dealers know who the other dealers are. So he takes out the opposition.
>
> (drug squad officer)

The same possibility is described by Pritchard in his 'no honour among thieves' version of informants. Pritchard was warned by his colleagues about the crafty buggers who talk because they want to increase their own turnover and profits. When they tip you off, it's because they want a rival off the street so they can pinch his business.

(Pritchard and Laxton 1978: 47)

Information from such sources is said to be rare but it can potentially be extremely valuable, because of the informant's intimate knowledge of drug dealing, and the wish to facilitate the police in eliminating the competition (Williams and Guess 1981: 239).

'Hell hath no fury'

Pritchard, a former undercover officer, was involved in a number of well-known cases including those of Howard Marks and Operation Julie. But there were less glamorous jobs as well. Describing his work using informants he identifies ex-girlfriends of traffickers as potential informants.

[A] good source of information was birds. That saying about hell hath no fury is dead right. If a drugs dealer breaks up with his chick, he had better watch out. The chances are that she will squeal, and we weren't too fussy how the information arrived.

(Pritchard and Laxton 1978: 46)

However, even in the days of 'birds' and 'chicks' there was some equality between the sexes, since Pritchard adds, 'Mind you, a bloke will do the same thing and for the same reason' (*ibid.*).[25]

There are also tip-offs which are motivated by a desire for revenge but which, in missing their intended target, reveal a new one. Pritchard recounts an example of this when some people just arrested threatened recrimination against the suspected informant. They named a man who they said they believed to be the informant, incorrectly as it turned out, and the police went and arrested him as well (*ibid.*: 49).

THE HANDLING AND PROTECTION OF INFORMANTS

Informants are probably the most important source of leads for the police, particularly in making drug cases. Informants' leads are often 'orienting' devices, telling the police which way and where to look. But they can be a lead to a great deal more, especially if the informant becomes a regular source of information and acts as a participating informant. But they have to be carefully cultivated if they are to be of continuing value. This is done through the inter-related exercises of *handling* (controlling) and *protecting* informants.

The Drug Enforcement Administration (1982: 65–8) manual suggests that informants can be controlled by an individual officer or by the commander of a unit who would then assign an informant to a detective. The former is preferable because then officers feel they are being given responsibility for controlling their informant; it avoids contradictory demands being made on an informant; and, perhaps most importantly, it enables trust and even friendship to develop between the informant and the detective. Williams *et al.* (1979: 38–9) found that most informants prefer to work with a single agent and the personal relationship that can be built up is akin to 'ownership' of individual informants.

At regional and local levels in Britain, most police forces have an Informant Registration System, which is run according to guidelines established by the Home Office and ACPO. The typical procedure might be that a drug squad officer working with an informant would notify knowledge of the informant to a Field Intelligence Officer (FIO), who can be sometimes part of the drug squad, otherwise outside it. The information is evaluated by the FIO and by a senior officer, and in turn this will be used to 'build up a picture' so that the original drug squad officer can assess the reliability of the informant and the information. All available information about an informant is put onto an intelligence sheet by the FIO and then passed on to whichever department is deemed to be most relevant. As one officer put it to us, 'Everything to do with informants is recorded. Each informant's got quite a thick file at the end of the day, so there's a lot of stuff there'. In one county force, an FIO outside the drug squad compiles 'target files' in cooperation with the targeting system of the Regional Crime Squad. The value of this system is said to be that all the 'donkey work' is done for the operational officers. The files are then evaluated by the officer in charge of the drug squad when and if the informant works with them. Some officers in other forces do not believe that this is necessarily the best system because the senior officer needs to get to know the informants so that the information about and from the informant can be evaluated directly.

Protecting the informant

Protection of informants is particularly acute around record keeping. The Drug Enforcement Administration (1982) says that both for reasons of alleged unethical and possibly illegal behaviour between the police and informants, and to maintain secrecy and protection of informants, the names of informants should be kept in one central file, with as few people as possible having access to it (see also Fuqua 1978: 177–8). In Britain, access to records on informants is strictly controlled so that, for example, an officer would not be able to discover the identity of other officers' informants simply by requesting that information. This safeguard means that criminals would have to corrupt an officer actually working in the appropriate records section in order to discover the identity of potential informants. The drug intelligence files kept in computerised form at the National Drugs Intelligence Unit (see Chapter 9) do not include the identities of the informants who supply much of the information on 'targets' and their associates.

In operational matters, one method of protecting an informant is for officers to act as if naive. For example, on a search 'Quite often when you are following up information, you know where to look but mustn't give your informant away' (Pritchard and Laxton 1978: 51).

In court the main element in the protection of informants is the refusal by the police to disclose their sources. In the American parlance, revealing the identity of an informant in court is quite eloquently known as 'burning' an informant. As this terminology makes clear, 'burning' is to be avoided whenever possible since the informant becomes useless as such thereafter, and may also require police protection. An obvious strategy for the defence then is to insist that if the defendant is to receive a fair trial the defence lawyer must be able to test the credibility of the police informant in open court. Usually the police will work on the presentation of a case in a way which does not reveal the presence of an informer, or rely on the established rule that the identity of informants will be protected in court.

In cases where the defence does manage to come close to evoking evidence about informers, a case will generally be dropped. For instance, in February 1989 Vincent Agar was sentenced to eighteen months' imprisonment at Teesside Crown Court after being found guilty of possessing amphetamines with intention to supply. Agar's defence was that the informant X had played a role in fabricating the case against him. X was said to be anxious to help the police because he was on a suspended sentence and in danger of going to prison. However, the judge prohibited defence counsel from asking questions of the police which might reveal X's identity (Herbert 1989: 21; Tan 1989: 16). On appeal in July 1989 the conviction was quashed.

> The Court of Appeal said that although there was a special and well-established rule of public policy which inhibited the disclosure of the identity of police informants, there was an even stronger public interest in allowing a defendant to put forward a tenable defence in the best light. The court said that the trial judge had erred in ruling that the defence could not put questions to police witnesses which might lead to the identification of the police informer.
>
> (Seton 1990: 3)

The Agar ruling influenced the case of John McPhee who was on trial on charges connected with the possession and supply of cocaine. McPhee pleaded not guilty and his defence was that the drugs had been planted on him by the informant. The judge said that he was bound by the Court of Appeal ruling in the case of Agar that if the defendant (McPhee) was to have a fair trial the informant would have to go into the witness box. The Chief Crown Prosecutor, in consultation with the West Midlands police, said that the informant's life would be endangered if his identity became known and consequently it was decided to drop the case (Seton 1990).

That non-appearance in court is one of the strongest elements in the protection of informants is confirmed by Wilson (1978: 71–2) who quotes an officer saying, 'All the informant wants is not to testify'. This officer had established and benefited from a reputation as being skilled at keeping his informants out of court: 'Word gets around if you don't burn 'em, and they'll work for you'. The 'working life' of an informant is most influenced by the skill used by the police in protecting them (Moore 1977: 164; Williams and Guess 1981: 241; also, on the range of protection measures, see Williams *et al.* 1979: 37–8; and on disclosure of an informant's identity, see Raezer 1987: 54–64).

The scope of corruption

Informants as described here are very much the 'bread and butter' of drug policing and informant leads are the mainstay of a number of operations. But as we have seen this relationship can also be a difficult one for the police, in the light of allegations about and instances of corruption (Cox *et al.* 1977).

Although corruption has been noted as a widespread problem in drug enforcement and does not relate only to informants, here we concentrate on the informant-related parts of it only. For Skolnick (1984: 123) it is 'the structural requirements of the narcotics enforcement pattern', including the dependence on informants, which lead to corruption. Skolnick (1984) argues that the enforcement pattern of 'working up the ladder' (which he says has limited utility) creates room within the organisation for wide discretion to be given to narcotics officers. One of their 'cultural axioms' is to protect their informants and this means that information has to be held back from superiors. 'As a result, the *opportunities* for corruption are *always* there and *always* a problem' (*ibid.*: 124, emphasis in original).

Skolnick then locates the potential and scope for corruption as arising from the structure and specialisation of narcotics enforcement (Skolnick 1984: 125–6; see also Manning and Redlinger 1978). Another thesis is that it is illicit markets themselves which generate opportunities for corruption, sometimes the systematic corruption of entire enforcement agencies (Kleiman 1989: 30).

Probably the most extraordinary recent case – and still the subject of allegation and counter-allegation – is that concerning the relationship between an informant and a senior Scotland Yard detective (Jennings *et al.* 1990). The context was the allegedly widespread corruption at Scotland Yard (Cox *et al.* 1977) such that, 'By the early 1970s the armed robbers were working the streets of London with impunity, assaulting banks, security trucks and Hatton Garden jewellers, seemingly at will' (Jennings *et al.* 1990: 31). The response at the Yard was an apparently wholesale move towards the 'supergrass' system of persuading criminals to turn in evidence against their colleagues. But while 'The policy did put many of the robbers in prison; it also guaranteed freedom to some of the worst offenders' (*ibid.*: 32).

It was in this climate, where there were significant rewards to be achieved by both informants (now virtually with a licence to 'run free' in exchange for information) and ambitious police officers (who could make major cases through a particularly good informant) that the relationship is said to have developed. Roy Garner was a known criminal with connections in armed robbery, VAT fraud and cocaine dealing. Tony Lundy was an officer in the Metropolitan Police Flying Squad. It is alleged that the relationship between the two men led to a situation in which Lundy became known as one of London's most successful policemen, while Garner received reward money on Lundy's recommendation as the source of information.

> In the space of three years Tony Lundy became the star detective at Scotland Yard. His declarations from the Old Bailey witness box of 'a war against crime' were headlined by the press. . . . At one trial after another he saw armed robbers given long jail sentences and then went off to relax with Roy Garner at the Torrington pub or the boxing club.
>
> (Jennings *et al.* 1990: 42–3)

In 1980 Garner was investigated by Met detectives in Operation Albany. Jennings *et al.* (1990: 68–77) say that although the investigators believed they had a 'cast-iron' case against Garner, they were told that Garner was a major informant, and no charges were brought. Lundy was investigated after allegations by another informant; an internal Scotland Yard report described him as 'corrupt' but the report was effectively covered up (*ibid.*: 102–3).

Garner is said to have become involved in the drugs business in the early 1980s. In this regard he is classically the type we have described as diversifiers in Chapter 3.

> When the 1980s dawned, Roy Garner was as quick as every other gunman in town to see that the golden age of armed robbery had passed. New types of crime beckoned and the professionals moved effortlessly into massive tax frauds and drug dealing. The temptations were overwhelming. . . . There were big sentences for drug trafficking but the use of couriers made for relatively small risks.
>
> (*ibid.*: 105)

The story as told by Jennings *et al.* (1990) is as follows. The fact that drug importation is largely policed by Customs and not the police was apparently ignored by the 'complacent' Garner. He started dealing in kilos of cocaine through a retail outlet, but eventually set his sights on a very large importation job. Around 1984 Garner learned that a Florida-based man was looking for European partners in cocaine smuggling (*ibid.*: 115). The man in Florida was Nikolaus Chrastny. Garner is said to have given Lundy's name as a reference to Chrastny and to be at pains to assure Chrastny that his 'police contacts would take care of things' (*ibid.*: 121). Chrastny bought 38 kilos of cocaine from the Medellin cartel in Colombia and – because they were said to be very keen on opening up the European market – they let him take another 354 kilos on 'credit' (*ibid.*: 123).

In 1986 a boat sailed from Panama to England; an exchange of goods took place off the coast and a second boat landed with 392 kilos of cocaine. An American investigation into money laundering started to uncover this cocaine conspiracy and with the investigation closing in on him – as well as a never transmitted BBC TV 'Brass Tacks' programme about him titled *The Untouchable*[26] – Garner decided to become an informer again (*ibid.*: 147). In October 1986 he met two senior Scotland Yard officers and told them about the importation of 710 kilos of cocaine in July 1986 (*ibid.*: 150–4). *The Untouchable* was remade for Granada TV's 'World in Action' series and transmitted in November 1986. It revealed the Garner–Lundy relationship and the fact that Garner had been the informant on the money laundering from the £26 million pound Brinks-Mat bullion robbery (*ibid.*: 154–6). South Yorkshire police were called in to investigate the programme's allegations.

Chrastny and Garner were arrested by Customs officers, although the former later escaped from Dewsbury police station in bizarre circumstances (*ibid.*: 167–8; Kirby 1989a:5). At his home, Lundy received a phone call from Garner's wife in which she passed on a message from her husband that he 'needed some help' (Jennings *et al.* 1990: 165). Lundy was suspended from duty immediately afterwards. The South Yorkshire inquiry submitted reports to the Metropolitan Police, the Police Complaints Authority (PCA) and the Director of Public Prosecutions in 1987/8. In August 1988 the PCA announced that Lundy was not to be charged with any crime but would face three disciplinary charges.

The most serious charge was headed: 'Internal Enquiry into Leak to Confidential Informant.' It stated that Lundy had 'communicated to Mrs Roy Garner information which you had as a member of the police force: in that you told her that she could tell her husband that certain information had been passed at a very senior level from Scotland Yard to senior personnel of the agency dealing with the case' . . . Now . . . Lundy stood accused of . . . passing on confidential information about the investigation into the cocaine conspiracy to Roy Garner.

(*ibid.*: 171)

The disciplinary hearings were not to be and in December 1988 Lundy was retired from the police on medical grounds (for his view on this, see Lundy 1989: 1,574). Garner's trial was in January 1989 and prosecution witnesses testified about his relationship with Lundy. In March 1989 Lundy appeared as a defence witness but most of his evidence was heard in closed court. The jury found Garner guilty of involvement in the conspiracy to import 392 kilos of cocaine and he was sentenced to 22 years' imprisonment (Jennings *et al*. 1990: 183; Tendler 1989: 5; Leigh 1989: 3).

The Lundy/Garner case is possibly unique in terms of the scope of corruption related to large drug importations in Britain. But there have been other examples which illustrate how fine is the line between cordial relations with an informant and corruption. Two recent cases illustrate some of the difficulties. Detective Sergeant Harrington, commended twenty-three times, appears to have fallen foul of a Metropolitan Police computer entry which questioned his honesty and his suitability for a secondment to the specialist criminal intelligence wing at New Scotland Yard. Sergeant Harrington's difficulties seem to relate to the case of Adrian Millar at Snaresbrook Crown Court in 1988, who was charged with possession and conspiracy to supply heroin. Millar had provided Harrington with information about drug dealing in the music business in 1982 and later appeared as a prosecution witness in a drugs case at the Old Bailey. Millar again provided information to Harrington when Operation Bridport in 1988 led to the seizure of a large quantity of heroin and the conviction of five defendants. Harrington appeared at Millar's case at Snaresbrook and told the court of the assistance that Millar had provided in at least two operations. Millar was found not guilty of conspiracy and the jury failed to agree on the possession charge. At Millar's second trial Harrington again gave evidence and Millar was acquitted (Hilliard 1989: 2,537). The officer clearly believes that the fact that he appeared at the trial of one of his informants has in some way been counted against him (*ibid.*).

Another case is that of Commander Roy Adams, a former head of the Metropolitan Police's criminal intelligence section, which arose after allegations made by a man arrested in a drugs raid (Cook 1990: 3; *Police Review* 1990a: 166). After a three-year inquiry by the Police Complaints Authority into allegations that he took bribes and had improper relations with criminal informants, the DPP decided that he had no case to answer.

Whatever the standards of integrity of individual detectives, they know that their relations with informants are amongst the most sensitive issues they will have to deal with and potentially lays them open to allegations of impropriety. We now turn to what is perhaps the most difficult area of enforcement.

STINGS AND SELLS: SOME CONTROVERSIAL TECHNIQUES

> The Government considers that police and Customs officers should not in any circumstances counsel, incite or procure the commission of a crime and cannot agree to change the guidance given to the police on this matter. Nevertheless, there may be scope for giving further guidance on which types of operation are and are not permissible within this rule, and the Home Office will consider this possibility.
>
> (Home Office 1990e: 12)

In this closing section we are concerned with some techniques that attract particular controversy because they involve either participating informants and/or undercover officers offering to supply or actually supplying drugs to their 'targets'. This type of operation is recognised as taking place in the US (Warner 1990: 1–5), where they are sometimes called 'stings'. It was the official position that no such operations took place in Britain at the time of writing.

Sell operations need to be distinguished from 'buy operations' – which are acknowledged to occur in Britain. As we have seen in Chapter 6, in a buy operation, undercover officers may attempt to 'work up the chain of supply' by posing as potential buyers. They may then attempt an immediate arrest at the time of the exchange ('buy bust'), or they may use the transaction to build up further evidence and make an arrest of this or a related trafficker at a future time (a more extended 'buy operation').

In a sell operation, by contrast, an officer or an informant offers either to sell drugs, or to put a potential buyer in touch with someone who could sell, or provides a sample of what it is suggested could be available for sale, or actually sells a consignment of drugs. This can then lead onto an immediate arrest of the other party ('sell bust'). In some cases, officers offering to sell a consignment never progress to the stage of actual payment, because the 'bust' occurs before the exchange of drugs and money is completed, the targets then being charged with conspiracy or a similar charge.

Alternatively, the officer or informant may simply use the offer of sale, provision of sample or actual sale in order to gain trust, stay in situ, and develop intelligence for use in the longer term. These are called *extended* sell operations. Typically, the sell proceeds and the target is allowed to leave the site of exchange, with officers holding back in order to achieve some other, more valued, objective on another occasion.

We now describe a range of such undercover operations, beginning with a 'sting' which targeted not a trafficker but a user.

Stinging the consumer

In the now notorious Marion Barry case a prominent black politician, the Mayor of Washington, DC, was persuaded by a female 'companion' to repair to a hotel room and there partake of a pipe of crack. A police video camera in the room recorded this consumption resulting in a controversial court case. Barry's defence was that he had been the victim of an FBI 'sting' operation, designed to discredit him politically. This claim was given added weight by the allegation that the US Attorney-General was personally involved in reviewing the plan for the sting operation (McNichol 1990: 12–13; Pringle 1990: 10; Tisdall 1990: 6). It was suggested that the 'sting' was an attempt by the authorities to record a spectacular success in the supercharged 'war on drugs' led by William Bennett, against the mayor of a city which Bennett had said lacked commitment to his war (Tisdall 1990: 6).

The case was heard in the full floodlight of media attention. The jury failed to agree on twelve of the fourteen charges against

Barry, finding him guilty only on one charge of cocaine possession at another hotel,[27] and acquitted him of the charge of possessing crack at the time of the 'sting'. The verdict was seen in some quarters as an object lesson on the unacceptability of 'sting' techniques when mounted against drug users, as distinct from traffickers. Nevertheless

> Federal investigators have no intention of abandoning the occasional use of 'sting' operations to make arrests in significant drug investigations, even though the tactic may have offended several of the jurors in the recently ended trial of Washington DC Mayor Marion S Barry Jr. . . . An 84-minute videotape of that planned encounter, ending in the Mayor's arrest, clearly showed the Mayor taking two separate puffs on a pipe during a visit to the hotel room of a former girlfriend, Hazel Diane 'Rasheena' Moore, who was cooperating with the FBI and local police at that stage of Barry's investigation. That kind of use of an illegal drug is normally more than enough [in the US] to support a possession charge. But the Vista [Hotel] count was one of 12 charges on which the jury could not agree. . . . On the charge emerging from the Vista Hotel sting, one juror has since told news reporters that the jury was split 6 to 6 – a clear indication, according to the juror, of doubts about the credibility of Ms Moore as a witness and about the government's motives in aggressively pursuing the whole case against the mayor.
>
> (Denniston 1990b: 1)

Thus, a carefully planned sting operation went wrong because the police failed to appreciate that convincing a jury is a moral task as well as a technical one, and that what can seem like 'bad behaviour' by the police can lead the jury to overlook law-breaking by the defendant. Such closely orchestrated sting operations can, depending upon the predisposition of jurors, seem to approach too closely the cruder tactic of 'planting' drugs on a target just before or during arrest.

In Britain, as in the US, there has in recent years been a considerable revival of interest in ways of policing the drug user (in addition to traffickers). Some argue that the law or guidelines to enforcement agencies require amendment to support sting and sell operations. However, we know of no advocates of their use in relation to simple possession (for personal use) in Britain. Nevertheless, the Barry case illustrates the potential of such methods of incriminating users. And in more mundane circumstances, given the shock likely to be felt by many of the people who might be caught in this situation, it seems possible that some at least would opt to 'put their hands up' and plead guilty in a lower court, rather than risk a contested case and heavier sentence in a higher court. This is a possibility that might be borne in mind by anyone tempted to advocate sting operations aimed at users.

Sell bust

These operations involve undercover officers or participating informants offering to sell or actually selling drugs to a person who they believe is a trafficker, then making an immediate arrest. It should be noted that such operations are generally brought to an arresting conclusion before any actual transaction takes place, thus obviating the need for informants or officers to trundle around with large quantities of illegal substances in their possession. Prosecutions may be brought on charges such as racketeering (in the US) or criminal attempts (a possible charge in the UK under the Criminal Attempts Act 1981).

In some cases, things are relatively straightforward in legal terms, because the unfortunate trafficker has unwittingly recruited a participating informant to deliver the drugs (either as a supplier, or simply as a helper/carrier) and so there is no suggestion of inducing the targeted person to break the law. The informant is simply informing the police of something that would probably have occurred anyway. The basis of this type of sell bust operation is for the informant to go along with the trafficker's plans, whilst police mount surveillance and move in at a convenient time – generally in a manner that either allows the informant to get clear first or to 'escape' in some convincing manner.

Difficulties can arise where the informant turns to the police for advice as to whether or not she should proceed. In this case the danger for the police is one of being drawn into what might possibly amount to a conspiracy that a third party, the targeted trafficker, should commit the offence of possession with intent to supply. The potential consequences might well run from the collapse of the prosecution case, to prosecution of the police. As the following quote from a drug squad officer illustrates, most experienced officers are alive to the dangers.

Of course the first thing that strikes you [is that] you are dealing with dealers, fingering the other dealers. When he [the participating informant] goes in there, taking in a parcel, delivering it . . . and then gives us the signal [that] the gear's in there. Now that's a big danger. It is a tremendous danger because what is happening there is an outright set-up, and although the officers concerned may be completely innocent of it, if it comes out in court to that extent it stinks to high heaven that a police officer got him to do that. Which is something that frightens the shit out of me every time I have a participating informant.

It is to safeguard against such difficulties that the police are careful to avoid giving certain forms of direct advice to their informants, and are careful to say nothing that could retrospectively be construed as instructing or encouraging them to 'set up' traffickers by causing them to possess drugs. The essence of a successful sell bust operation is that the motivation for the sale of drugs by the participating informant or undercover officer to the would-be buyer must be seen to come from the latter.

We have been told that some officers explain the potential problems to the informant so that the informant will not put them in an embarrassing position by asking the officer whether to set up the target. Rather, the informant who wishes to cooperate to a high degree with the police simply informs the handler that s/he intends to follow such a course of action or is thinking of doing so. If the officer strenuously and convincingly objects, then the informant desists. But if the officer does not object – or does so apparently without conviction – then the informant may well go ahead, telling the officer details of times and places.

In such cases, the police would probably be free of any impropriety in law. After all, there is no over-riding obligation upon the police to prevent each and every criminal act; if by letting one criminal act occur and arresting the miscreants a series of offences can be prevented, then arguably the public interest has been served.

'Licensed dealers'

A type of undercover operation that we identify with certainty as occurring in Britain at the present time is that involving an informant who, with or without the knowledge of the police, continues to deal. Some police officers acknowledged that some of their informants might continue to ply their trade, and we heard the same thing from informants.

> You know, you can say 'I'm a licensed drug dealer!' Because your CID [Criminal Investigation Department] officer knows that you've learnt to do these little things [and says] 'As long as you don't have a disorderly house and you don't have any category A drugs in your house, you carry on doing that and we'll make sure you're all right, you just keep telling us who's doing the burglaries, where the cheque cards are going'.
>
> (police informant)

So, a locally known identity as a petty trafficker provides a reasonable cover for an informant who passes to the police information not only about other traffickers but also about other criminal activities. Additionally, in the US at least, trafficker-informants are occasionally used to help officers to identify the buyers in an area. By selling relatively small amounts but making oneself available as one who may later be able to supply much bigger amounts, trafficker-informants put themselves in the position of being approached by other traffickers who wish to obtain large amounts (possibly because their other means of supply are temporally unavailable).

Sells and 'exchanges'

Another technique, which we have no reason to believe occurs in Britain, is used to trap a dealer in Class A drugs. Here the police draw out some cannabis from police stores. An undercover officer then approaches the dealer in Class A drugs and offers, in 'exchange' for the Class A drug, half the value in cannabis and the other half in money. This is regaled as particularly useful since it allays the dealer's fears about entrapment, since they 'don't expect the police to be selling to them' (drug squad officer). In Canada, we are told, this technique is considered acceptable because it leads to the arrest of a dealer in Class A drugs in exchange for the 'sale' of a Class B drug (cannabis).

Intelligence development through extended sell operations

We turn lastly to the undercover officer offering to sell drugs to traffickers who, it is judged, cannot be cornered by a buy operation or other means. This is without doubt the most sensitive area of drug enforcement in Britain, with as much public keenness to deny current involvement as there is private keenness to get support for such operations in future.

The lack of support for such operations at present stems from two sources. First, it reflects anxiety that sell operations would infringe the law on incitement, breach of which would not only cause the case to be thrown out of court but also lay officers and the police force open to prosecution. Second, it reflects a confusion between sell bust as such and the more subtle use of sells, without arrests at that time, as part of a wider intelligence development operation. In Britain, sells occur only as part of a carefully handled and extended operation in which any subsequent arrests occur in apparently disconnected circumstances. One basis for prosecution then involves evidence *other than* the sell. To the defence this might appear suspicious in hindsight – but, lacking proof of incitement, do they really want to drag evidence of past transactions into court, further incriminating the defendants? Such, at any rate, was the gist of the accounts given us by officers who confirmed the existence of a limited number of extended sell operations in Britain, stating that such operations had been authorised in certain circumstances.

Extended operations – both buys and sells – are also being used to develop intelligence about other matters, related to drug dealing, such as money laundering. The use of financial instruments such as futures and options, bank drafts and insurance pay-outs constitutes an expanding area of crime which US and British investigators are keenly following. Extended sell operations provide one means of penetrating these financial transactions.

Finally, these extended operations, without arrests of traffickers or money launderers, provide an opportunity to develop strategic intelligence – defined in Chapter 9 as getting a much broader view of what is going on, for example how any particular market is developing. We believe that this much longer-term aim underlies some of the extended operations now occurring.

Such confirmation as we have been able to dig out has been hedged around with qualifications. It will be interesting to see if a more open discussion about such methods will be forthcoming.

We believe that a public discussion of such techniques of law enforcement – which of course have potential applications not just in relation to drug trafficking but in many other areas of criminal law – should precede their introduction in practice. Unfortunately, an informed and reasoned discussion does not seem to be within the remit of the Home Affairs Committee, where Members of Parliament might have been expected to show serious interest in questions of the boundaries of legitimacy in enforcement matters. Following crack panics that spread from the US to Europe in late 1989 (Home Affairs Committee 1989a; *Druglink* 1989), there were behind-the-scenes pressures for a relaxation of the restraints on sell bust in Britain. The Home Affairs Committee (1989b), in a muddled passage, said

> We are not convinced that the drugs problem can be tackled entirely by traditional methods of law enforcement. . . . We note that the [Home Office] Minister did not appear to rule out the possibility of officers purchasing drugs from dealers . . . since that would not be playing a prominent part in inciting the dealer's crime.
>
> (Home Affairs Committee 1989b: xxix)

This is patent nonsense, since it is very clear – and not denied by anybody in drug enforcement – that buy bust is alive and well in Britain, as witnessed by successful prosecutions (see Chapter 6). The Committee incorrectly lumped together buy bust with sell operations (which are officially denied). In these pages we have tried to provide a more adequate account of the present situation, as far as this can be known.

CONCLUSION

In view of the general argument throughout this study, sell operations, their use in the US and their uncertain position in Britain, are very significant for our understanding of the drug market.

They show that the 'work up the chain' type of buy bust operation has its limitations in practice – some of these limitations being determined by the security-consciousness of traffickers. But the greater and inherent limitation of trying to work up the market is that its validity as a strategy depends on a notion of a flow of drugs passing through stable and downwardly branching conduits, from big trafficking operations to small.

In reality, however, the structure of the market is much more fluid and people's positions within it tend to change. Someone who is trafficking at one level of the market (e.g. in kilograms) at one time may be acting at another level (e.g. grams) at another time. Also, someone who at one time wishes to sell may at another time have a potentially big buyer or several buyers and yet be short of the commodity required. In these circumstances any over-reliance on buy bust in an attempt to get 'the big traffickers' must fail – as the historical example of the DEA shows (Wilson 1978). The interest in sell operations is an implicit recognition that the shine is coming off the 'big trafficker' mythology.

A new control mix is emerging in which enforcement attempts to hop 'across' and 'down' market as much as 'up' market. These developments can be seen as going hand-in-hand with so-called 'demand reduction', emphasising policing drug retailers and their customers (Bennett 1989; Warner 1990), as a symptom of disenchantment with the mythology of trafficking.

Within this context, the use of informants seems set to increase. Initiatives such as offering larger rewards may, in retrospect, come to be seen as a relatively forgettable aspect of 1990s drug enforcement. What seems more likely to be the legacy is the increasing numbers of petty traffickers and users swept up in the net, some of whom will be induced to give information in return for suggestions of an easier disposal. It would be wrong to say that once an informant, always an informant. Nevertheless, there seems little doubt that after acting as an informant on one occasion, the relationship with the police thus struck up does increase the chances of a repetition. It seems, therefore, that the expanding field of drug enforcement provides one channel of more general social surveillance and social control (Marx 1988). In Chapter 9, we examine the centralisation and full computerisation of the agency that will handle and, increasingly, direct this enormous workload.

Chapter 9

Intelligence rules
The centralisation of policing in Britain

> Criminal Intelligence can be said to be the end product of a process often complex, sometimes physical and always intellectual derived from information which has been collated, analysed and evaluated in order to prevent crime or secure apprehension of offenders.
>
> (ACPO 1975: 7)

This may be the first use of the term 'intellectual' in a high-level British police report. The British police traditionally have not seen themselves much as intellectuals (indeed, as the popular mythology goes, the first intellectuals involved in policing were amateurs – the Sherlock Holmes and Hercule Poirot types). The 1980s, however, have witnessed the rise of the intellectuals in the police, and nowhere more so than in intelligence, which, leaving aside anti-terrorist measures, meant especially drugs intelligence.

Just as detective work in earlier decades became an elite within policing, so intelligence work is increasingly seen as a desirable stepping stone in the career of clever and ambitious officers. Whoever defines 'intelligence' defines the whole direction of enforcement. Intelligence is becoming the tail that wags the dog. The tendency for operational matters to be strongly influenced by and, to some extent, actually *directed* by intelligence priorities, is emerging and, we suggest, likely to grow in the 1990s.

So, what is intelligence?

INTELLIGENCE: STRATEGIC AND TACTICAL

'Intelligence' is a very slippery thing to define. One of the few points of agreement is that intelligence is not the same as information, but is a processed form of information.

A simplified but adequate approach recognises that information and the process which can convert it into intelligence are essential to operational planning.

(ACPO 1986: para 1.8)

Here we have an information > processes > intelligence > action cycle, with the emphasis upon the processes whereby information may be transformed into that guide to action that is called 'intelligence'.

The question of the nature of those transformational (intelligence-producing) processes is, we suggest, best asked in relation to the type of action that is envisaged. Conventionally, action may be at the level of overall *strategy* (what to do about crack on the eastern seaboard of the US), or at the level of *tactics* (how best to reduce open-air dealing in a particular street) (cf Drug Enforcement Administration 1982: 88; Lawn 1985). Strategic and tactical intelligence can be distinguished on three criteria: time-scale, verifiability and politicisation.

Time-scale

Strategic intelligence is concerned with long-range predictions of the development of a problem, and with the overall effect of particular enforcement strategies on that development; whereas tactical intelligence (sometimes called operational intelligence) is concerned with the next few months. The collation of strategic intelligence suits those whose forte lies in selecting out diverse forms of information and fitting them into a theoretical model of what is going on on a broad front (e.g. 'cocaine has reached saturation point in the US'). The collation of tactical/operational intelligence, on the other hand, suits individuals and small groups who thrive on putting information to fairly immediate use.

Verifiability

By its nature, the quality of long-range strategic intelligence is difficult to assess, since the feedback period is long and it becomes difficult to disentangle the various causes and effects; whereas, with the short timespan of tactical/operational intelligence, it is relatively easy to verify through action (one can find drugs or not). Hence, for example, when in Britain a crack cocaine epidemic seemed slow in arising, in spite of urgent DEA warnings of its coming, everyone claimed credit. Those who had adopted the DEA view claimed that it was their quick response which averted the problem, whilst those who suggested that the British context made for different drug problems also preened themselves.

Politicisation

All intelligence is constructed by the sifting out of some types of information and the search for other types, according to the criteria laid down for intelligence. (For example, the Regional Crime Squad targeting system, described later in this chapter, encourages collection of information relevant to intelligence about certain types of targets.) However, although all intelligence-making is selective, strategic intelligence-making is by its nature more open to political considerations. Hence, for example, cocaine intelligence is developed in strategic and tactical forms, whereas amphetamine and its precursors are foci for tactical intelligence operations, with less interest in the broad strategic picture. We hear little about amphetamine 'flooding' Europe, yet it is a more widely available stimulant than cocaine.

Clearly, the transformational processes involved in collecting information and turning it into strategic intelligence are rather different from those involved in turning information into tactical/operational intelligence. Although it would be wrong to over-do this distinction (it is certainly not a dichotomy), there are differences between the ways in which intelligence work is done at a national and local level.

US drugs intelligence and foreign policy

The history of the development of drugs intelligence in the United States has been a relatively 'top down' one, at least ever since 1969 when President Nixon designated international narcotics control as a concern of US foreign policy. Nixon set up a 'White House Task Force on Heroin Suppression'. There followed the establishment of an Office of Narcotics Coordinator in the Central Intelligence

Agency (CIA), particularly orientated towards the development of strategic drugs intelligence (Bamford 1983: 325). The CIA worked with the Bureau of Narcotic and Dangerous Drugs (BNDD). Because the BNDD lacked authorisation to intercept communications within the US, it was assisted by the National Security Agency in this regard (*ibid.*: 327–8).

Throughout the Nixon era there was a struggle between the security agencies and the White House on the one side, and elements of Congress and the Judiciary on the other, on the legitimacy of the activities of the intelligence agencies – which included active interception of the electronic communications of thousands of people in the US and abroad (*ibid.*: 380). The legitimation of this extensive surveillance apparatus has, in various turns, been the internal security of the US in relation to communists and fellow travellers, the anti-Vietnam war and student organisations, civil rights and more militant organisations and, finally, drugs. In 1972 a Presidential executive order established an Office of National Narcotics Intelligence within the Justice Department, aiming to develop a 'National Narcotics Intelligence System' to carry through what Nixon described as the 'total war against dangerous drugs' (*ibid.*: 332–3). This formed the institutional and cultural context within which the Drug Enforcement Administration formed in 1973 by a merger of the BNDD and several other enforcement agencies (Wilson 1978), and the FBI, the two agencies mainly responsible for drug enforcement, generate their pictures of the world. Since these agencies are part of the wider intelligence community, it is not surprising that strategic drugs intelligence is generated in a manner compatible with the broader policy objectives of the United States.

It takes only a little historical sense to perceive the consequences. Strategic intelligence about priority drug problems has been quite closely related in the post-Second World War period to aspects of foreign policy. During the 1960s and into the 1970s, when the US was embroiled in the Far East, the illegal drug most closely associated with that region, heroin, was the focus of enforcement efforts (and also of some covert US government agency involvement: McCoy *et al.* 1972; McCoy 1974). At that time, it should be recalled, cocaine was widely regarded as a relatively benign drug, comparable to cannabis as a recreational intoxicant. By the 1980s, however, with its Far Eastern burden unhappily resolved, the focus of foreign policy concern shifted to

South America and, in this context, the dangers of cocaine – a product primarily of that continent – were sharply re-evaluated. At the same time, the domestic debate over problems of the inner city, and the hardening of political attitudes and enforcement responses to drugs and crime generally, helped to keep the issue of cocaine trafficking at the top of the policy agenda. Thus, from the 1960s to the 1980s, cocaine displaced heroin as the drug of greatest concern.

The foreign policy-linked context of the construction of strategic drugs intelligence may provide quite some scope for it to be detached from tactical intelligence (information about what is actually happening on the ground). Such is the stress put upon the value of strategic intelligence in the US that in his 1990 Drug Control Strategy the President called for an entirely new drugs intelligence centre, within the Department of Justice, to produce a strategic picture 'of how the drug war is to be fought' against 'international drug trafficking enterprises' (*Drug Enforcement Report* 1990a: 3). The definition would seem to exclude domestic production of drugs. The Senate Appropriations Committee, acting on criticisms that a new and separate unit would only add to the confusion and 'turf wars' that characterise US drug control, blocked funds for the new centre. But another Senate Bill passed in July 1990 authorised $150 million of funds confiscated from traffickers to be spent as the President's Office of National Drug Control Policy sees fit in 1991 fiscal year (*Drug Enforcement Report* 1990c: 1). Thus the new strategic intelligence centre could be set up from 1991 onwards, entirely separate from the existing El Paso Intelligence Centre, which has hitherto had both strategic and tactical intelligence functions.

History of British drugs intelligence

In Britain, there seems less likelihood of strategic drugs intelligence dominating tactical drugs intelligence (although the DEA-inspired crack panic of late 1989 shows the scope for distortion). Partly, this may be due to the fact that the history and structures of British drugs intelligence derive mainly from a *ground-up process* in which, originally, detectives generated their own intelligence and then began to specialise in making it available to others. Criminal Intelligence in the police can be said to have commenced in the early 1950s with the formation of the C9 Branch at New Scotland Yard. Primarily it was formed as a liaison department to assist enquiries by provincial officers in connection with the investigation of country house break-ins thought to have been committed by London criminals . . . in the late 1950's it was realised that to successfully combat organised crime and to achieve the apprehension of prominent criminals, efforts would have to be made to accumulate as much information as was humanly possible regarding such individuals. . . . In consequence it was decided, with Home Office approval, to form a Criminal Intelligence Branch at New Scotland Yard . . . [followed by similar bureaux in Birmingham, Cardiff, Durham, Glasgow, Liverpool and Manchester.]

(ACPO 1975: 1)

The regional bureaux were later to evolve into today's Regional Criminal Intelligence Offices but the bulk of intelligence collation continued to be done in London. There, various *specialist* intelligence units subsequently evolved – reflecting the historical, quasinational role of the Metropolitan Police in providing specialist services that may be used by other British police forces. In 1973, partly as a result of 'a crisis of confidence' following revelations of corruption in the Metropolitan Police drugs squad, the Home Office and ACPO intervened to transfer the files of that squad to a new Central Drugs and Illegal Immigration Intelligence Unit (Grieve 1987, vol 1: 175).

The combination of drugs intelligence and immigration intelligence reflected a perception (which recurred in the 1980s) that it was immigrants, legal and/or illegal, who were responsible for much of the importation of illegal drugs into Britain. In this respect Britain differs from the United States, insofar as in the US drugs intelligence was rather more linked with national security and anti-communist concerns, than with race and immigration. In 1984 the Central Drugs and Illegal Immigration Intelligence Unit was re-designated the Central Drugs Intelligence Unit. This broke the direct organisational linkage between police drugs intelligence and immigration intelligence (though this resurfaced as 'Operation Lucy', later re-formed as the Crack Intelligence Coordinating Unit, targeting Jamaican people). In August 1985 the Home Office appointed a National Coordinator for Drugs Intelligence. As a civilian employee, the National Coordinator oversaw the transition of the Central Drugs Intelligence Unit (staffed by the Metropolitan police) to a National Drugs Intelligence Unit (staffed by police drawn from all major forces and by Customs, with neither in the ascendancy) in November 1985.

At regional level, drugs intelligence has tended to be more integrated into broader criminal intelligence, rather than being such a specialist or separate intelligence activity. Regional Crime Squads (RCSs) set up from 1964 to deal with serious crime were followed by 'the setting up of Criminal Intelligence branches in each region' (ACPO 1975: 2), handling drugs alongside other forms of intelligence. Although the RCSs subsequently developed specialist *operational* 'drugs wings' as recommended by the 'Broome report' (ACPO 1985 – see Appendix), drugs *intelligence* did not evolve into a separate system at regional level, perhaps partly because of the relatively low level of trafficking outside London before the 1980s.

So, historically, the organisation of drugs intelligence in Britain has been influenced in the direction of specialist drugs intelligence by the Metropolitan Police's assumption of a quasi-national role (leading to the establishment of the Central/National Drugs Intelligence Unit in London), but Chief Constables representing police forces outside London have tended to favour integration of drugs intelligence into broader intelligence systems. In spite of the availability of political backing during the 1980s for high profile and by implication specialist responses to trafficking, the balance of opinion within the Association of Chief Police Officers has favoured integration. As a succession of reports shows, ACPO's expert and considered assessment has tended to be that the relationship between trafficking and other crimes is close enough to merit integration of intelligence functions. Thus the 'Baumber report' (ACPO 1975) saw integration of intelligence functions as the way forward at national level and suggested the setting up of an integrated national criminal intelligence office. This recommendation was repeated more firmly a decade later by the 'Ratcliffe report' (ACPO 1986), which also foresaw the 'integration of the National Drugs Intelligence Unit into the [proposed] National [Criminal] Intelligence Office' (ACPO 1986: para 6.7; Home Affairs Committee 1990).[28]

Ratcliffe also perceived the existing pattern of management of Regional Crime Squads and Regional Criminal Intelligence Offices as providing a model for management of a national office: 'It is recommended that the Standing Committee of Chief Officers currently responsible for the overview of the

RCSs assume a similar role in respect of the [proposed] NIO [National Intelligence Office]. The NI [National Intelligence] Coordinator could then report to this committee' (1986: para 6.9).

This in essence was the solution subsequently adopted by the Association of Chief Police Officers (ACPO) in July 1990 (*Police Review* 1990d: 1,478; senior intelligence officer interview 1990). The Home Office was expected to accept the recommendation and to sort out funding in time for the Coordinator of the National Criminal Intelligence Office (or Unit, Centre or Service) in 1991, becoming fully operational from 1992 onwards.

This development illustrates two trends in British drugs intelligence: first, to build up intelligence systems (for both drugs and crime) from a local and regional level upwards, rather than top-down; and second, to incorporate drugs intelligence into an enhanced system for handling all criminal intelligence (drug and non-drug, strategic and tactical/operational). On the latter point, as the Baumber Report had earlier pointed out in relation to local intelligence databases – and as is equally true at national level – a lack of integration of databases undermines the purpose of intelligence. 'It allows, for example, information on a person retained in one system dedicated to drugs problems to be totally isolated from information on the same person which is recorded in another system dealing with general criminal matters' (ACPO 1975: para 4.4). The National Criminal Intelligence Service will use the new computer coming into use from 1992, Police National Computer 2, on which it will be possible to search across records of all types.[29]

The consequence of the two rather different histories of drugs intelligence in the US and Britain is that, whereas in the US strategic intelligence considerations tend to shape tactical intelligence (e.g. in relation to domestic concerns about Latin America, cocaine, etc.), this is to a lesser extent the case in Britain.

TACTICAL INTELLIGENCE IN BRITAIN

What is good intelligence, as far as operational drug squad officers are concerned?

In an endeavour to find out what [police] officers thought was 'good' and 'useless' intelligence, respondents were asked to give example of each, illustrating their point wherever possible. From their replies we were able to extract the following variables:-

Intelligence that is current and detailed	35.7%
Intelligence that is corroborated	23.3%
Intelligence from a tried and trusted source	18.8%
Intelligence that has a high evaluation score	17.0%
Intelligence that proves right on investigation	15.9%

(Waymont and Wright 1989: 49)

For historical reasons, the concept of intelligence held by operational officers is closely linked to 'information received' from established informants (see Chapter 8). Given this history, the perceptions of officers as reported by Waymont and Wright are perfectly comprehensible: good intelligence is up to date, detailed, comes from more than one source, comes from people in whom one can place some credibility and proves right on investigation. That only one-sixth of respondents mentioned the last aspect indicates that although officers are of course interested in intelligence that is accurate, they acknowledge that some intelligence might be uncheckable and not lead to an immediate operation, yet still be useful for background.

The development of a national focus for drugs intelligence in Britain in the 1980s involved considerable controversy in police and Customs circles. Rather predictably, given the rivalry that existed at the time, there were suggestions by the police (ACPO 1985: 41) that Customs cease to use its own, independent database, called CEDRIC, for recording drugs intelligence, and use the police's then Central Drugs Intelligence Unit (CDIU) instead. Equally predictably, Customs did no such thing, but the subsequent evolution of the CDIU into the National Drugs Intelligence Unit (NDIU) did see the two services working together in the one unit (under a nominally civilian head, with two deputies, one from each service). HM Customs and Excise kept their own drugs database. Additionally, just as the police at lower and middle levels of the force structure keep more information on card indexes and sometimes on microcomputers, so Customs also keep much of their intelligence on microcomputers (Waymont and Wright 1989: 61). Nevertheless, the NDIU has developed apace and forms the basis for an integrated National Criminal Intelligence Service.

A national intelligence service

At the NDIU, tactical drugs intelligence is recorded centrally on computer under three main headings: Target description; Associates (of the targets); Free text (commentary). The procedure is for an officer in the field to telephone the NDIU and to brief a member of NDIU staff, who inputs information to the computer under those headings. Entries may run to scores of 'associates' and many pages of 'free text', giving extensive information about the target.

Much of the information forwarded to the NDIU comes from informants and, partly for this reason, there is a need for users of that information to have an estimate of its worth. The key point is to establish the likely reliability of the information, so that it can be assessed as 'intelligence'. The Association of Chief Police Officers has agreed standard criteria for the assessment of the reliability of informants and their information (ACPO 1986) and this is routinely used at local and national levels. The two-part grading system consists of a *source code* and an *information code*. There are four source codes:

A – where there is no doubt about the authenticity, trustfulness and competence of the source; or if information is supplied by an individual who in the past has proved to be reliable in all instances.

B – is the grading given to information from a source who has in the past proved to be reliable in the majority of instances.

C – is the grading for information from a source who has proved to be unreliable in most instances in the past.

X – is for information from a previously untried source.

The source codes are complemented by accuracy-defining information codes, based on the proximity of the informant to the information being supplied:

1 – is for information known to be true without any reservation.
2 – is when the information is known personally to the source, but not known by the reporting officer.
3 – when the information is not known personally to the source but is corroborated by other information already recorded.
4 – when the information is not known personally to the source and cannot be corroborated. (ACPO 1986: Appendix C)

This coding system relates closely to Williams *et al.*'s (1979) work which indicates that the quality of information is central to the police's enforcement activities. The reliability of the source has to be complemented by the reliability of the information and, 'In general, the more specific the information, and the more that can be corroborated, the greater its credibility' (Williams *et al.* 1979: 36–7; cf the evaluation table in Williams and Guess 1981: 242).

It is difficult to draw any conclusions about how well informant coding systems work in practice: what gets recorded must be open to a degree of variation. There is a well-acknowledged temptation for individual officers to keep to themselves information that they may be able to use to good effect later, rather than passing everything on to other officers and to the NDIU.

Intelligence ownership and sharing

A central intelligence database would at first sight appear to be sensible and unproblematic. But there are in reality a great many problems with the workings of the system, the first of which is whether or not officers are sufficiently motivated to send their intelligence in to the centre.

There are conflicting signs about the extent to which the NDIU receives sufficient high quality intelligence from field officers. On the one hand the Broome Report stated that 'the Unit is now in the position of having a surfeit of high quality intelligence. This surfeit revealed a dearth of operational capacity to use it' (ACPO 1985: 36). Similarly, whilst we were conducting our research, we noted quips from operational officers along the lines of 'don't worry, we don't want to know about your informants, we've already got more intelligence than we can deal with' (drug squad officer). On the other hand, there was a near-consensus that operational officers are sometimes loath to share high-quality intelligence, preferring to keep 'nice jobs' for themselves. Others have noted this tendency.

> Intelligence sharing between police units and between police and other agencies was reportedly limited, although in some places a higher degree of mutuality came from personal relationships of trust. In the worst examples we heard of, cases were aborted rather than passed to another unit or agency. Again, and we do not apologise for repeating this point, much of the resistance to the sharing of intelligence can be ascribed to the way in which output is measured and judged, including assessment for career purposes. All detectives will recognise these attitudes as part of the detective ethos but unless they are modified there is little prospect of improvement in intelligence sharing.
>
> (Waymont and Wright 1989: 61)

In 1989 the NDIU's Coordinator, giving evidence to the Home Affairs Committee, referred to the problems of intelligence sharing and to two possible ways of improving intelligence flows.

> One of the solutions – and I put this hopefully as a short term solution – is that we can develop a national criminal intelligence system. Another way in which improvements can be made is that it comes right down to the question: who owns intelligence? At the moment I have to use all my persuasive powers and my staff do to get people to deposit intelligence into the unit. I think if we wish to address and attack this problem then *there ought to be some authority that I can not only ask for but demand*. I believe in that way we could produce better intelligence for the operational people in the field to be more effective.
>
> (Price 1989: 123, emphasis added)

Our own discussions with officers in Regional Crime Squads and other units suggest that the extent of intelligence sharing may vary over time and across the country. One RCS officer declared that

> We use NDIU a lot. Our management stick to the guidelines. Some forces won't use NDIU. I think that this really dates from the time when drugs weren't a problem, and then there was kudos in keeping a secret [because a significant drugs arrest was rare, whereas today it is commonplace], but that generation of officers has nearly gone.

As this illustrates, operational officers at regional level are generally prepared to forward their intelligence to NDIU. There is no real disincentive to do otherwise, so their self-perception as professionals working with other professionals motivates them sufficiently.

On the other hand, officers lower down in the system may have at least two disincentives to sharing intelligence. First, the lower down in the hierarchy one is, the more likely that one's intelligence will be lost on the way to NDIU, because someone further up the chain does not understand it or think it important enough to forward. Second, there is the possibility that an operational unit higher up in the chain would take over the bigger and potentially more interesting jobs if they knew about them. Some of the counter-measures adopted by local officers were quite creative. For example, we had described to us cases where, coming across an 'importation job', drug squad officers got directly in touch with Customs and formed a coalition with them, jointly pursuing the target. The joint operation was then declared to NDIU, in circumstances in which a higher-level operational police unit would be unable to take over the job. We heard of gnashing of senior officers' teeth in such circumstances. But the danger for officers and squads adopting such courses of action would be that such short-term successes are achieved at a price, which could be blocked promotion (not something that would unduly worry drug squad officers happy in their present work), sideways re-assignment out of drugs work (which would worry many), or rapid promotion out of drugs work (a form of approbation that can generate ambivalent feelings).

A related problem to that of refraining from sharing intelligence has been that some officers learnt to use the NDIU database as a means of erecting a formal boundary fence around 'their jobs'. The way in which this was done is called, in NDIU parlance, 'flagging'. Up until 1990, any officer could protect any number of potential targets from investigation by other officers, simply by notifying those targets to NDIU and asking for them to be flagged in his or her name. Other officers who subsequently enquired about any flagged targets would then be warned to leave them alone. The rationale of the flagging system was the prevention of different squads tripping over each other in relation to any given target. However, the system laid itself open to abuse: officers could protect targets even more effectively by flagging them than by failing to notify them to NDIU in the first place. From 1991 onwards, this will be reduced by new NDIU procedures.

> What was happening before was we were passive and people were saying we've got an interest in this person and people were being less than honest, were protecting what I call their proprietorial right in an individual by flagging [the case]. We weren't daring to ask them why. But now, given the coordinator's key tasks and our terms of reference to coordinate operational activity, what we now say is that before anybody can flag something they have to demonstrate that there is a dedicated operational team or intelligence team looking at and dedicating resources to that operation so that we can protect their rights. Now that will mean that instead of a squad of a hundred men having a hundred operations which is one operation per man which is totally unrealistic we could expect [a large drug squad] to have twenty target operations which might have four or five different targets within it. So we're being much more assertive.
>
> (senior intelligence officer)

Such measures alone might be expected to reduce field officers' motivation to forward their intelligence to the centre. Compensating this, however, are new restrictions on the extent to which intelligence forwarded by an officer can be revealed to another without the permission of the originator.

> What we will now say to people [enquiring subsequently about those targets] – and this is with the agreement of the police and Customs – is 'Yes, we do have information [about that target] and somebody will be in touch with you'. And then we go back to the operational officer [who originally introduced that target into the system] and say, 'What do you want us to do? Are you going to tell him or are we going to tell him?'
>
> (*ibid.*)

It is anticipated that these changes will both prevent excessive ownership of targets by operational units (it being the national intelligence centre that will 'own' all intelligence) and also reassure officers that the intelligence that they contribute will not be disclosed to other officers without good reason.

The willingness to forward intelligence to the centre may or may not be enhanced by organisational changes that are made possible by the shift from a paper records system, to an integrated computer-based system. On the plus side, the shift to a single computer means that operational officers working at regional level will at least know that their information will in all probability get straight on to the national database, rather than being lost, discarded, or diverted sideways into a paper system by regional-level intelligence officers who are responsible for sifting and passing on intelligence as appropriate. In the system as it will operate from 1992

> What's going to happen is that there is going to be a National Criminal Intelligence Office [at the top] and there's going to be branch offices. . . . Regional Criminal Intelligence Offices will go, and they will become branch offices of the NCIO. The NCIO will set the policy . . . [and] will be responsible for all of the issues, for the type of records that will be kept. These branch offices will be responsible for the criminals resident within their area who are committing crimes of the nature that we are interested in, cross-border and regional crime. When it lifts itself up above a region into a national and international arena, the NCIO will be responsible for the ownership of that record.
>
> (senior intelligence officer)

Clearly, if bureaucratic structures and rules are seen as determining police behaviour, then the balance of ownership of knowledge is tilting from the operational detective to the national intelligence officer. There are other ways in which this balance may be tilting, too. In thinking about this, what cannot of course be predicted is the long-term response of people in the field.

Intelligence packages

Alongside the long-running debate within the police about intelligence and who, if anyone, 'owns' it, there has been an equally lively debate about 'intelligence packages'. At issue here has been the question of whether or not it is realistic to expect a national intelligence unit to develop directive operational plans which could be forwarded onto local and regional operational units to enable them to initiate new operations in appropriate ways.

This idea is linked to the expectation, formed in the 1970s, that intelligence units should show particular interest in 'establishing the identification of a particular individual when a *series* of crimes is being committed' (ACPO 1986: para 4.1), since 'the ability to recognise a *crime series* is a prerequisite of coordinating police resources to maximum effect' (*ibid.*: para 1.10). The underlying concept is that past patterns of crime can give a steer to the deployment of policing in ways that anticipate future offences. Such an approach is obviously most likely to be applicable in relation to those individuals and organisations who are already known to the police as career criminals, offending over an extended period of time (typically, the diversifiers whom we described in Chapters 3 and 6).

During the late 1980s there was some expression of dissatisfaction within the police over the failure of the NDIU to provide such intelligence packages to operational teams. Locally based officers complained with irony that, having telephoned the NDIU for information on possible targets in their area of operation, often all they got back was the information that they themselves had submitted. Responding to such criticism, the NDIU's Coordinator distinguished between the prospects for proactive intelligence in relation to local drug seizures, and in relation to precursors (chemicals used in the manufacture of drugs such as amphetamine) and money flows.

I know that criticism is levelled that the Unit does not provide intelligence packages. I just do not know what an intelligence package is in their [the critics'] terminology. To me an intelligence package is where you have a full intelligence service which can hand something over to an operational team directing them to go to this address at this time and find these drugs and those people. If those are the aspirations of the people in the field they are ignorant of the intelligence process and a lot of them are. That is just not achievable on a regular basis. We are already giving out intelligence packages of a sort through the precursor monitoring section. I do not wish to describe in detail how that unit functions but we are able to point investigating teams to areas of work where they can *develop* the intelligence we have into a successful operation and discovery of a laboratory. Also in the financial section we are receiving information on banks and other sources and we *develop* that within the Unit by searching across other information/intelligence that we hold so that we are able to pass that on to an operational team, giving them a very good start on the road to an investigation.

(Price 1989: 127, emphasis added)

The drugs intelligence system then had to some extent become a victim of its own success, its claims having raised expectations beyond its ability to deliver – in respect of intelligence in its operational sense. Breaking out of this cul-de-sac necessitated an attack on the old definition of *drugs* intelligence. The three types outlined in Price's statement – precursor monitoring, financial investigations and intelligence development (national direction of local operations) – are described in the remainder of this chapter. Between them, these three aspects of the intelligence system constitute the ascendance of this function of policing over the more familiar, substance-focused, operational side.

NEW TYPES OF INTELLIGENCE

Following the chemicals: precursor monitoring

Precursor monitoring is considered one of the growth areas of drugs in intelligence. Interpol defines precursors in the following manner.

> A precursor chemical is a raw material that is specific and critical to the production of a finished chemical, product. . . . The term 'immediate precursor' is usually applied to precursors which are only one reaction step away from the final product [whereas] . . . Essential chemicals are less specific or critical than precursors to the production of the final drugs, and usually have widespread legitimate industrial applications.
>
> (ICPO General Secretariat 1989: 19)

Interpol go on to note that

> Placing these chemicals under international control similar to drugs is not a viable solution because of the enormous quantities used in legitimate manufacturing processes. In addition, although national restrictions on chemicals may be imposed, experience shows that they can be circumvented easily when supporting measures are not imposed by other nations. The most effective strategy may be . . . an international programme of selective monitoring and exchange of information.
>
> (*ibid.*: 21)

This is an area in which the Commission of the European Communities (CEC) is claiming competence as regards chemicals crossing frontiers. A draft Regulation, following the spirit of Article 12 of the Vienna Convention (which covers control of precursors) foresees that

Each member state shall take, in accordance with its legal system, appropriate measures to encourage operators to immediately notify the competent authorities of any circumstances, such as unusual order and transactions of scheduled substances [twelve are mentioned in an appendix], which indicate that such substances destined for import or export may be diverted for the illicit manufacture of narcotic drugs or psychotropic substances.

(Commission of the European Communities 1990)

As both Interpol and the CEC draft regulation makes clear, compulsory monitoring of all transactions in precursors is not regarded as realistic. Most European countries have a voluntary system. In Britain, the NDIU has a section specialising in this. The aim of precursor monitoring is summed up in one of the NDIU's objectives.

To maintain a database on manufacturers/suppliers of precursor chemicals and other substances/articles used in the illegal production of drugs in the UK and elsewhere; act as the focal point for the liaison arrangements with manufacturers and suppliers and to support operational units with intelligence and other data held centrally.

(NDIU no date)

Initially, in the early 1980s, the NDIU wrote to 3,000 chemical companies in the country, collating outline information on their sales of over 200 chemicals. The list was then narrowed down to just under 1,000 companies producing those chemicals most likely to be used in the production of illegal drugs (NDIU sources). The list of chemicals concerned is confidential but it would be surprising if it did not include acetic anhydride (used in heroin manufacture), ephedrine (for methyl amphetamine), methylamine and safrole (MDMA or Ecstasy), and methylamine and potassium permanganate (for cocaine manufacture). All chemical companies are said to cooperate in a voluntary scheme based on the idea of 'profiling'. A buyer profile raising suspicion might be: purchase of a chemical on the short-list; a new customer; an unknown company name; a cash sale; and, for some chemicals, an export order to a developing country. In such cases the chemical company voluntarily notifies a Home Office official, who passes on the information to the NDIU, who in turn alert operational teams to investigate.

Precursor monitoring has had its successes. In Operation Washington, a London-based chemical company responded to an NDIU enquiry, saying that it had someone interested in buying ephedrine, which is used to make methyl amphetamine. The potential buyer, Walker, had claimed to be involved in a battery acid business. Police records identified him as a small-time villain who had some years before been linked to the illicit purchase of benzyl methyl ketone (BMK – an amphetamine precursor) but no legal proceedings had followed. Walker paid by cheque for £8,000 worth of ephedrine, but the company was suspicious, even though ephedrine can be used in the battery acid business. A police check on Walker's letterhead showed that it had a bogus VAT number for the business. A financial disclosure revealed that his account had only very recently become over £20,000 in credit. When Walker arrived at the chemical company and took possession of the ephedrine he was followed by a Metropolitan Police Area Drug Squad to an address in Kent. After surveillance at that address the chemicals were seen to be moved to an isolated cottage. There a number of people wearing respirators and overalls were seen to pour petrol on a number of containers and set fire to them. A subsequent search by the police revealed traces of methyl amphetamine and ephedrine in the remnants of the fire. Now certain that they had identified a laboratory, the Area Drug Squad continued its surveillance operation on the men, who were observed moving a consignment to a lock-up garage. A warrant was obtained to search the garage where seven and a half kilos of 89 per cent pure methyl amphetamine was found. Another fifty kilos of ephedrine was also found to be stored there. The white powder was replaced with another product by the police and a surveillance operation continued on the garage. There was then pressure on the police to curtail the operation due to its high cost, particularly once the seven and a half kilos of methyl amphetamine had been uncovered. However, the surveillance continued and the substitute white powder was seen to be loaded onto a truck and transported northwards on the motorway. The truck was stopped on the motorway and eight people were arrested. Forensic evidence was used to tie in these people with the methyl amphetamine. Subsequent searches produced various manufacturing equipment and utensils from which an estimation could be made of the amount that the group had been involved in making. Two of the group were said to have admitted their involvement in the production of methyl amphetamine, and other chemicals found suggested that up to 150 kilos of methyl amphetamine was to be produced. Chemical profiling of the drug suggested that little had been sold on in the UK (i.e. 'street seizures' had a different chemical 'signature'), and that most of it was destined for the United States. (On methods of chemical profiling of drugs see Barnfield *et al.* 1988: 107–17.) Subsequent police enquiries arising from the questioning of suspects led to the pursuance of monies said to be held in banks in Gibraltar and the US.

The complexity of this case means that the actual investigation moved from precursor monitoring to surveillance to something like 'controlled delivery' (substitution of the drug) and then finally on to financial investigations, in order to substantiate the conspiracy allegations against a group of nine men, while three others were extradited from the US to stand trial in Britain. Six people were convicted.

The monitoring of BMK has been a productive source of tracing the factories where drugs are manufactured. As one NDIU officer said to us, 'In 1982 when we first started monitoring BMK [benzyl methyl ketone] . . . first of all the results were tremendous . . . it took them five years to realise that BMK was being monitored'. Other examples of the productivity of 'following the chemicals' include a check on a Dutch company buying 500 litres of BMK. The company was found to be falsely declaring its reasons for buying the chemical; this led to an operation against the firm by Dutch police and an estimate that they could have been linked to the production of between 2,000 and 3,000 kilos of amphetamine per year. Of the six laboratories detected in a nine-month period in 1989, two were uncovered by conventional police methods and both were said to be small-scale amphetamine laboratories. All of the remaining four were discovered through monitoring of precursor chemicals – an amphetamine factory had ten kilos of the drug, a methyl amphetamine factory led to the seizure of fifteen kilos of the drug, and an MDMA manufacturing site led to the seizure of 100,000 tablets (the first seizure of such drugs in the UK).

The results of precursor monitoring can potentially be spectacular in cases like Operation Washington and the ones described above (see also Tendler 1988: 3). Two reservations should be noted. One is that precursor cases need not be complex or involve targets at a particular level of the market. They can be relatively routine operations, leading to the netting of little more than minor user-dealers, albeit ones actually doing the manufacturing themselves. As we saw in the case of a Regional Crime Squad in Chapter 5, a routine follow-up of sales of a particular chemical led the RCS to a lone buyer manufacturing amphetamine for personal use and some sales.

Secondly, hailed as it has been as an important source of intelligence, precursor monitoring has had its problems. In Britain, monitoring of the amphetamine precursor BMK began in 1982, but amphetamine manufacturers soon became aware of this and began to make BMK themselves from other chemicals. By 1987, the number of laboratories identified dropped from over ten a year to three, each of them being identified by means other than precursor monitoring (NDIU officer). As the authorities moved on to the precursors of BMK ('essential chemicals', in Interpol parlance; ICPO General Secretariat 1989: 19), independent sources suggested a displacement effect.

> The speed scene seems to have fallen apart. There's very little speed around. What is around is ephedrine, you know there's an awful lot of ephedrine being sold as speed, unknown to users and sometimes to quite big dealers. One of the reasons one suspects for this is that big dealers have moved on to methyl amphetamine or on to Ecstasy. That's where the money is. And there is difficulty in getting some of the precursors for making amphetamine sulphate – apparently its's much easier to make methyl amphetamine. . . . Once you shut one door, people move to another.
>
> (Andrew Fraser, personal communication 1989)

The drug market is often described as a squishy balloon: squeeze here, and another bit bulges out there. If precursor monitoring has had any hand in shifting the market from amphetamine sulphate (generally snorted) to methyl amphetamine (generally injected, or in the crystalline form of 'ice', smoked), then this must at best be regarded as a mixed result. No doubt precursor monitoring has a big future in drugs intelligence, but this can be an unambiguously positive future only if used selectively to shape the market, rather than in the expectation that it or any other measure can stop it in its tracks. Which are the manufactured drugs that we would most like to see displaced, and which other drugs would we be prepared to see around in larger quantities in their place?

Following the money trail: financial investigations

While precursor monitoring is an important development in drugs intelligence, financial intelligence has a much broader significance within the criminal justice system. Financial investigations may have two functions: they provide new avenues for beginning drug trafficking investigations, and they are the basis upon which the proceeds made by convicted criminals are assessed by courts and hence determine the confiscation order to be imposed after sentencing. (The Drug Trafficking Offences Act 1986 is discussed in the next chapter.) Both functions are facilitated by financial disclosures by banks and similar institutions. Here we focus on the ways in which financial investigations open up new avenues for beginning anti-trafficking investigations.

Because of the international nature of the banking system, reciprocal agreements between countries to cooperate in cases crossing frontiers have been entered into. By 1990, Britain had such agreements with Canada, the Bahamas, Australia, Bermuda, Switzerland, Spain, Anguilla, Nigeria, Gibraltar, Malaysia, Sweden and other countries. Financial investigations are handled at three levels: at the national level, by a Financial Section in the NDIU and by Customs officers; at a regional level, by designated officers in drug profits confiscation teams attached to the Regional Crime Squad drugs wings; and at a more local level in some major cities, notably London, by smaller specialised units. There were 1,274 financial disclosures in relation to drug trafficking made in Britain in 1989, double the 1987 and 1988 figures (*Drugs Arena* 1990: 15). Two-thirds of these disclosures were made to Customs, one-quarter to the Metropolitan Police (whose central drugs squad is expected to become the drugs wing part of an RCS) and the rest more or less evenly spread over the country. It should be noted that disclosures are also made in relation to the Criminal Justice Act 1988 (covering any gainful crime) and additionally, the Prevention of Terrorism Act 1989.

Financial investigations begin in one of two ways: first, a financial institution may approach the authorities because they have noted a transaction in the account of a customer that seems out of place, or second, a financial investigator may approach a bank with a request about a particular customer's account (having grounds for suspicion that that account may be involved in drug money transactions).

In the United States, the Bank Secrecy Act 1970 places an obligation upon banks to notify the US Treasury within fifteen days of *any* deposit of money in excess of $10,000 (Dorn and South 1990). As Zander notes in a wide-ranging review of the US law relating to drug trafficking, this Act

> has not made much, if any, contribution to law enforcement. One problem has been that not all banks have complied with the requirement. Probably it is the least reputable that are the worst offenders. But even when the banks do comply, the benefits seem slight. One state regulator said that the reports simply gather dust since 'nobody knows what to do with them'. The General Accounting Office (GAO) said in a report in 1981 that few law enforcement agencies used the reports.
>
> (Zander 1989: 47–8)

A problem with this cash transaction reporting (CTR) system is that it produces a 'deluge of information' (*ibid.*: 48) which cannot be adequately monitored by the authorities. It is estimated that 8 million CTR forms would have been filed in 1990 (US SFRC Subcommittee on Narcotics and Terrorism 1990: 14). Both enforcement agencies and the banks in the US are said to recognise the value of the CTR system, with some of the former stating their usefulness in intelligence analysis and developing new investigative options. However, as the Subcommittee also notes, criminals have exploited the CTR system, and the backlog in analysing information it has generated, deliberately filing extra CTR reports (*ibid.*: 15–18).

In Britain, however, the system is a voluntary one based on the more sophisticated idea of profiling. In this context, a suspicious profile might be, for example, a large transaction through a quite new account; or an unduly large transaction for a particular account; or a transaction involving a country where drugs are produced or through which they may be routed. In such cases a clerk may report suspicions to a supervisor, who then discusses the matter with a manager. If the latter believes that there may be grounds for suspicion, then s/he will contact the local police, Customs or NDIU *without reference to the customer concerned*. In many cases, a bank will contact local police direct. NDIU enters the disclosure into its records and attempt to cross-reference it against any known or suspected 'target', 'associate' or other datum held in its computer system (see above).

Such information may then become a new element in an existing investigation or it may be the starting point for a new investigation. An investigation might involve checking through information obtained on fiche from Companies House, checking a company's returns, profits, and directors; looking at the pattern of trading and bank transactions over time; following up trading links to see if the company actually does the legitimate business it claims to do; checking with the Land Registry; checking with the Inland Revenue (drug squad officer). Section 27 of the Drug Trafficking Offences Act 1986 obliges any company to disclose its pattern of business with another company which is being investigated, and section 31 prohibits such a company from telling the suspected party about the inquiries. In one case, a bank clerk was jailed for four years for tipping off a suspected party.

The Irvine case illustrates one way in which a bank disclosure may initiate investigations. Irvine, a diversifier in the terms of this study, was known to the police as having a history of crime, but was not suspected of having any involvement in trafficking. Irvine's wife attracted attention by attempting to move £100,000 from a bank account, triggering a bank reference to a Drug Profits Confiscation Team. The team brought in operational officers who raided Irvine's premises and brought him to committal. They then attempted to construct a picture of his financial dealings going back over six years but found it difficult to sort out which money was drug related and which was not.

Similar problems have been experienced by other investigators where, for example, a sudden paying of a house mortgage may be the result of trafficking, or company fraud, or other financial crime. This difficulty has been reduced by the formation of Asset Confiscation Teams, following the passage of the Criminal Justice Act 1988, with the responsibility for tracing *all* criminal assets. However, the amount of work generated is 'a nightmare' (drug squad officer) and the only way to deal with it may be to involve operational officers more in asset-related work.

In another case, a previously known criminal called Miles bought a flat and paid £40,000 into his co-habitee's account. A clearing bank informed the NDIU, who told an assets team. Coincidentally the drug squad had Miles under surveillance. He bought a greengrocer's shop, leading drug squad officers to speculate that he might be 'retiring'. A year later, however, an informant told another detective unit that Miles was dealing, triggering a two-day surveillance operation and raid that yielded eight ounces of heroin.

Financial inquiries are particularly useful as an investigative tool in those cases when physical surveillance is difficult because the target is surveillance-wise (e.g. see Chapter 3) or the nature of the area makes it difficult, or there is insufficient police personnel power (surveillance being very time consuming and hence expensive). In some police forces, about half of all drug trafficking investigations may now be triggered off initially, or at least in part, by a financial disclosure by a bank or another financial institution. However, in other forces, informant-initiated investigations still form the majority of cases (interviews with Asset Confiscation officers). Whether such differences are due primarily to financial institutions varying in their willingness to make disclosures, or to the keenness and capacity of local enforcement units to process such disclosures, is unclear. What the trend may be as regards the future balance between financial disclosure-initiated investigations and informant-investigated ones, remains to be seen. However, surveillance will always be necessary in some cases, for example those when people do not have bank accounts because they deal in cash (Confiscation Team officer) and where they are involved in exchange or 'record-less banking', based on trust (NDIU sources; on 'Hawala' banking see *ICPR* 1989: 28; Devalle 1989: 9).

As the British courts fully take on their obligation to make a confiscation order in every case of conviction for drug trafficking – under the Drug Trafficking Offences Act (DTOA) 1986 – so the demand upon asset investigation teams will grow, since they are required to conduct an asset investigation *in advance* of the verdict. We have, for example, seen several cases in which an assets investigation is done for the court in respect of persons without any property, resulting in assessments that their proceeds from trafficking amounted to no more than a few hundred pounds. This is absolutely in line with the DTOA. But it is an onerous obligation on asset teams and is certain to reduce their capacity to process bank-initiated disclosures that might lead to new, often more substantial investigations being opened. Hence the potential of the DTOA as a tool of financial *investigation* may be undermined by its requirements on the financial *punishment* side. This is a point to which we shall return.

National intelligence direction of local operations

In July 1990, the Association of Chief Police Officers (ACPO) agreed a long-standing proposal for a National Criminal Intelligence Service, into which the existing NDIU will be absorbed by 1992 (*Police Review* 1990d: 1478). The proposal was swiftly accepted by the government. Indeed, one Chief Constable told us that the Home Office had been keen for the proposal to be agreed but had wanted the proposal to be seen to be ACPO's. Just as importantly, ACPO also agreed a proposal that the Regional Crime Squads provide an 'intelligence development' arm for the NCIO.

As discussed in the Ratcliffe Report (ACPO 1986), intelligence development is seen as falling in between 'operational matters' and 'intelligence gathering'. It means doing things in the field – sometimes going beyond surveillance to include covert operations – but stopping short of action such as raids or arrests. This is by no means a new conception of intelligence development, but the increasing importance accorded it and its increasing direction from the national policing agency has a potential significance much wider than drug enforcement. Regional Crime Squads, under the general direction of the Executive Coordinator of RCSs, follow requests of the national intelligence office to 'develop' specified intelligence leads.

Thus, in the context of changes taking place in British policing in the early 1990s, intelligence development implies a hiving-off of some of what used to be called 'operational' matters, redesignating these as an aspect of 'intelligence', to be done at the request of and under the general guidance of the national intelligence centre.

Together with the other changes referred to above, in particular the tighter control of all intelligence by the national centre, the emergence of nationally directed intelligence development shifts the balance of drug enforcement (and other enforcement) away from local and regional operational units, and towards the centre. So, rather than regional officers receiving intelligence packages ('go to address X and you will find a kilo of heroin') from the national centre, they will receive an intelligence development directive ('keep an eye on address X and tell us what you see'; 'get someone to visit and attempt to make a buy'). The resulting intelligence will be fed back to national level for assessment alongside intelligence from other sources.

The involvement of Regional Crime Squads (and their drugs wings) in intelligence development as requested/directed by the national office *implies* that, once involved in such a task, an RCS would refrain from 'going operational' without the agreement of the national office. There may be a number of other implications that are difficult to work out in the abstract, but will become clearer in practice. Overall, however, intelligence development looks like a Trojan Horse for the centralising tendencies that have marked British policing since the 1960s.

The Broome Report (ACPO 1985) raised some advantages of a national detective agency but noted the constitutional difficulty, which boils down to a concern that a national police force might involve accountability to the Home Secretary and hence to the government of the day. The NDIU, which was set up as accountable to the Home Secretary, was denied an operational capability for this reason. It has now, however, acquired the power to direct others to carry out operations. This means that the National Criminal Intelligence Service into which the NDIU will be absorbed by 1992, together with the Regional Criminal Intelligence Offices which will form its 'branches', and the Regional Crime Squads will in effect form one integrated intelligence development and operational organisation.

In effect, this is the national detective agency, debated as long ago as 1975 (ACPO 1975), expected date of birth 1992.

CONCLUSION

The development of drugs intelligence, precursor monitoring and financial intelligence are growth areas in law enforcement. It seems doubtful that, lacking the concerns about drug trafficking and use that surfaced so sensationally in the 1980s, these developments would have achieved the momentum they have. It is in this sense that this area of crime has been most 'productive': it has stimulated structural changes, helping to mobilise public support for trends that might in other circumstances raise a ripple of controversy.

Underlying all of this has been the European dimension. The threat of terrorists and drug traffickers being afforded easy passage within the new frontier-less Europe has also provided a powerful impetus to these structural changes in British policing (Imbert 1989; Home Affairs Committee 1990; Clutterbuck 1990).

There is a down-side to all this. There are clear grounds for concern from a civil liberties angle, especially in relation to some of the more sophisticated undercover methods that are being tested out well in advance of any public debate of them. And more broadly, we are moving into a period of expansion of social surveillance measures and intelligence databanks in which previously separately stored bits of information about citizens are being brought together (Marx 1988). This could be considered as being in the general interest if the system works fairly, for example hunting down corporate criminals and environmental polluters as eagerly as tin-pot drug traffickers.

The persistent structural problem in the British situation is the lack of democratic oversight. The National Criminal Intelligence Service, with considerable powers across the boulevard of law enforcement, will be answerable to a committee representing other interests within the enforcement community.[30] It will not be answerable to Parliament or to any other democratic body. Some readers will probably find such observations redundant. But we think that, given the range of powers to be exercised by the NCIS, discussion of its accountability needs to be put onto the public agenda.

Chapter 10

The punishment illusion
Your money *and* your life?

It is generally agreed that the powers afforded to the enforcement agencies are sweeping, and the sentences handed down by the courts are 'draconian' (Zander 1989). In Britain, persons convicted of trafficking face up to life imprisonment, plus confiscation of their assets if these are presumed to be the proceeds of trafficking.

Asset confiscation, as originally recommended by the Hodgson Committee, was intended to be a just but humane penalty. It would take away from convicted parties their ill-gained wealth, thus overcoming the perceived scandal that a person might serve a prison term and then be free to enjoy that wealth, as occurred in the notorious Operation Julie case (Hodgson *et al.* 1984: 3).

It had been envisaged that the imposition of a confiscation order would be 'taken into account in reducing the length of a prison sentence' (*ibid.*: 138). In the excitable anti-trafficker climate of the 1980s, however, this aspect of the Committee's recommendations was overlooked. The Home Office, in the knowledge of the likely recommendation of the Hodgson Committee, and in spite of being concerned about Britain's growing prison population, announced that maximum terms of imprisonment for drug trafficking were to be increased, and this was subsequently confirmed by the Controlled Drugs (Penalties) Act 1985. The Association of Chief Police Officers' Broome Report applauded that move (ACPO 1985: 60) although, in common with others calling for longer terms of imprisonment, it did not give any reason for doing so (cf Home Affairs Committee 1985).

The following pages put these developments in the context of the history of development of penalties in general, suggesting that trafficking legislation is very much the curate's egg of crime control.

DRUG CONTROL: THE STORY SO FAR

As far as crime control in general is concerned, there is now a considerable literature pointing out that increasing surveillance of citizens and situations has been a historical trend from the nineteenth century to the present day (Foucault 1977; Cohen 1979; Mathiesen 1980; Marx 1988). This has involved not just the creation of a public police, with access to increasingly elaborate camera surveillance and computer databases (public and private), but also the involvement of private security firms (in shopping malls, etc.) (South 1988) and, finally, the mobilisation of every citizen in *Crimewatch* programmes. Associated with this is

> a sharp increase in the number of registered crimes over the period in question (that is, not due to an increase in the detection rate, or other variable of that kind). The increase in registered crimes could be the result of (1) a real increase in crime; (2) an increased willingness on the part of the public to report crimes to the authorities; (3) an increased readiness on the part of the police to discover crimes on their own initiative, and not through the public reporting ('direct discovery'); or, of course, a combination of any two or more of these possibilities. . . . [I]t is probable that the main reason for the increase in registered convictions in the post-war period is *either* a real increase in crime, *or* an increased willingness by the public to report crimes . . . either way, the public is reporting more crime to which the social-control system has to respond in one way or another.
>
> (Bottoms 1983: 183–4)

To Bottoms's list of possible factors causing the increase in crime, we must of course add another – the creation of new categories of crime by legislation.

Drug control provides examples of this. Throughout most of the nineteenth century there were no controls on the production, sale, import/export or possession of drugs (other than laws regulating the circumstances of sale of alcohol – Dorn 1983). Some legislation did emerge in relation to the sale of medicines containing opiates (Berridge and Edwards 1981). It was not until the First World War and thereafter that the modern structure of narcotic controls began to emerge. Regulation 40B of the Defence of the Realm

Act 1914 made it an offence for anyone except doctors and similar professionals to possess cocaine, following alarm at reports that it was being taken recreationally by British troops. The Dangerous Drugs Act 1920, which was primarily motivated by the need to ratify international treaties, made it an offence to import, distribute or possess morphine, heroin and cocaine. The maximum penalty for any such offence was a £200 fine or six months' imprisonment for a first offence – a far cry from the multi-years' prison sentences to be imposed upon traffickers by the mid-1980s. In an interesting precursor of asset confiscation, the 1920 Act provided for a fine of £100 or three times the value of drugs that were imported or exported. That the legislation was not seen as effective can be judged from the fact that the Dangerous Drugs and Poisons (Amendment) Act 1923 increased the penalties to a maximum of £1,000 fine or ten years' imprisonment, but only when prosecution had the consent of the Attorney-General or Director of Public Prosecutions. Cannabis was added in the Dangerous Drugs Act 1925. Permitting premises to be used for smoking or dealing in cannabis was proscribed by the Dangerous Drugs Act 1964, and the Drugs (Prevention of Misuse) Act 1964 controlled amphetamines. LSD was controlled in 1966.

There was little change in the drug legislation until the Misuse of Drugs Act 1971 which, beside consolidating previous legislation and bringing Britain in line with post-war international conventions (Bruun *et al.* 1975), made the distinction in penalty terms between possession offences and supply offences. Modern thinking on drug control derives from debates of the 1960s which led up to the 1971 Act. Drug *users* became described as weak personalities, typically trapped in deprived environments, who had been led astray by misguided peers and unscrupulous drug pushers. They were sick or immature, and required treatment, counselling, or simply a safe space to grow as people. Drug *dealers*, on the other hand, come to be perceived as belonging to a quite different category. One word suffices to describe them: 'bad' and, as reaction hardened, 'evil'.

It was not until the 1980s that the concept of drug 'dealing' metamorphosed into that of drug 'trafficking'. During the 1970s, most Europeans referred to drug 'pushers' or drug 'dealers'. Anyone referring to 'trafficking' would have been regarded as rather quaint, the term seeming to hark back to nineteenth-century concerns with slavery. By the end of the 1980s, however, the term 'drug trafficking' had come into common usage, in the context of increased penalties and images of violence. A similar shift in language had occurred in the 1970s in respect of street crime, as the term 'mugging' crossed the Atlantic and acted as the linchpin of a wave of police/media/public fears about violent crime by young blacks (Hall *et al.* 1978). And it is clear that 'trafficking' has similar, albeit more extreme connotations, carrying definite implications of dangerous foreigners and a need for severe punishment.

However, the increasing focus upon traffickers as objects of surveillance and control has not left drug users unaffected. Repeated panics – about amphetamines and cannabis in the 1960s, heroin and solvents up until the mid-1980s, and cocaine and synthetic drugs in the late 1980s – have kept the spotlight upon drug users, especially when they are involved in small-scale supply. Whereas in earlier years such persons would have been described as 'user-dealers', today they become 'minor traffickers', and worthy of a considerable effort in bringing to court (cf Chapter 7).

The development of financial penalties

As regards punishment in general, the growth of the fine was noted earlier this century as occurring across Europe.

> Imprisonment remained the central point of the whole system, but it received increasing competition from the fine. . . . This phenomenon is not merely the result of new crimes . . . but is also the consequence of a general policy of substituting the fine for imprisonment.
>
> (Rusche and Kirchheimer 1939: 166–7)

Part of the explanation for the growth of financial penalties is evidently the expansion of the money economy to incorporate the majority of citizens. There is limited scope for the use of such penalties in a society in which a sizeable proportion of citizens have no disposable income and little property that may be seized and sold. It is clear that there are certain necessary conditions to be met before a criminal justice system can begin to switch from taking away liberty to taking away the money. The fine became increasingly common in a climate of increasing European prosperity, although

Even in England, the rise of the fine for adult indictable offenders has not been one of steady progress. The first great growth came in the late nineteenth century, but thereafter the proportionate use of the fine remained fairly static until the Second World War, during and after which there was a further increase in use. . . . There have also been considerable fluctuations in the post-1945 growth of the fine, with, for example, little increase since 1970.

(Bottoms 1983: 168)

The latest development of financial penalties is asset confiscation. Both fines and asset confiscation are now used, in addition to life imprisonment, for convicted drug traffickers. Asset confiscation was brought into British law by the Drug Trafficking Offences Act (DTOA) 1986. Asset confiscation means the confiscation of those assets of a person found guilty of an offence to the extent to which some or all of those assets may be suspected or shown to derive from crime (Dorn and South 1991).

Confiscation of the *proceeds* of crime generally goes wider than the *profits* of crime, since the latter phrase refers only to the difference between first, a criminal's investment in a criminal enterprise, and second, the proceeds from that enterprise. Under the DTOA, it is the whole of the proceeds (i.e. investment plus profit) that is subject to confiscation. This means, for example, that if a criminal extends his or her mortgage on the family home by £100,000 in order to finance a drug deal, and if s/he is able to sell the drugs on for £200,000, then the latter sum (and hence the house itself) is at risk, not the former sum.

In the case of a conviction for any trafficking offence, the court must make an order for confiscation of all the proceeds estimated to have been obtained not only from the offence(s) proved, but also from any other trafficking offence that the court believes may have occurred over the six years prior to when proceedings were instituted. It is not necessary for the prosecution to show that more than one offence was committed. Rather, and exceptionally in British law, the presumption is that any asset acquired over the past six years which cannot be shown by the defendant to have been obtained legitimately may be regarded as being the proceeds of trafficking, and confiscated. The burden of proof is reversed.

In these respects the DTOA follows the recommendations of the majority of the Hodgson Committee (Hodgson *et al*. 1984). However, a Note of Dissent by two members, Andrew Nicol and Clive Soley, objected to the concept that a person should have an order made against them for offences which were presumed, but not proven to have been committed.

> In our view . . . it is contrary to a basic principle of our criminal justice system to sentence a person for an offence that has not been proved or admitted. The other members of the Committee would empower the judge to resolve a disputed issue of whether the defendant were guilty of further wrongdoing. This is not satisfactory in our view. Defendants are entitled to have allegations of serious criminality resolved not by a judge but by jury and we fail to see why they should lose this right because they have been convicted of other, different crimes. The proposal is made apparently to save court time. Yet we do not see how this can be done without depriving the defendant of proper procedural safeguards.
>
> (Hodgson *et al*. 1984: 144)

Nicol and Soley go on to suggest that any reversal of the burden of proof would contravene the European Convention on Human Rights. Article 6(2) of the Convention states that 'everyone charged with an offence shall be presumed innocent until proved guilty according to law' (*ibid.*). However, a confiscation order under the DTOA does not amount to a finding of guilt in respect of presumed trafficking; it is simply a confiscation order. For example in the case of Jill (described in Chapter 2 and below), although found guilty on only one count, she was estimated by the court to have supplied several kilogrammes in the past. Accordingly, the court applied a confiscation order calculated on the basis of the street value of that larger amount.

If the convicted party does not pay the amount reckoned by the court to be the proceeds of trafficking, and if the court believes that they hold hidden assets or property outside the jurisdiction of the court, then an additional period of imprisonment is imposed by the court in place of the financial penalty. Failure to comply with a confiscation order results in additional periods in prison, according to the following scale.[31]

£10,000–20,000	12 months
£20,000–50,000	18 months
£50,000–100,000	2 years
£100,000–250,000	3 years
£250,000–£1 million	5 years
Exceeding £1 million	10 years

Thus it is possible for a person to be jailed for several years for presumed but unproven offences. In such a case, one is being jailed for failing to follow the confiscation order, rather than for the presumed offence.

If the court is satisfied that a convicted party is unable to raise the whole of the sum specified in the confiscation order – for example, because they no longer have possession of part or all the money received for the drugs sold, having spent the money on living expenses and/or luxury items – the amount confiscated is whatever remains (DTOA, section 32/4(3)). In Jill's case, the court estimated that the total proceeds of the drugs she sold in small lots over an extended period amounted to £2 million. But, since her available assets amounted to only about £30,000, that was the amount of confiscation order. Jill ran her life in a business-like manner, building up savings on the scale that any other self-employed person might expect, and on conviction she lost those savings. People known to her who were convicted at the same time had apparently spent their money. The law apparently creates an incentive for traffickers to lead an extravagant lifestyle since savings are likely to be confiscated upon conviction.

During the initial years of operation of the DTOA, some police officers voiced concern that the courts were failing to follow the full requirement of the Act, especially in relation to relatively minor trafficking offences. It was felt that traffickers who do small deals over an extended period of time generate considerable cash-flows. Other officers described the duty upon the court to make a confiscation order on every convicted party as onerous, both for the courts themselves and for the police. Specialist officers are tied up in preparing reports for all trafficking offenders, to be available to the judge in the event of conviction. Consider the situation of one offender.

The defendant does not have access to either bank or building society accounts, his living expenses being derived from his state benefit income. His rent is paid direct thus leaving a little over

£10 per week for general purposes. However when one considers his admitted drugs expenditure, he requires additional income in order to satisfy it as the profit from [drug] sales despite his admissions is not sufficient for re-purchase. A breakdown of cost and retail pricing is shown [in an appendix to the officer's report]. The defendant also states that he smoked cannabis himself. If he smoked the 104 grammes he purchased that would represent 416 cigarettes, therefore over a two week period, the period he states he would buy further supplies, he would have to smoke 29 cigarettes (joints) per day, which clearly his constitution would not tolerate. The prosecution therefore assumes that the £273 with which [the defendant] purchased the cannabis together with the £48 in his possession upon arrest represents the proceeds of drug trafficking and therefore invites the Court to make a Confiscation Order.

(from a Financial Statement prepared by an officer in a Drug Profit Confiscation Unit)

In this case, since the defendant had been assessed as having received £273 + £48 as proceeds of trafficking, yet had no realisable assets other than the £48 in cash, it was the latter which was taken from him. The financial cost, in terms of police investigation and court time, of making this order is not known. Some observers claim that the obligation for the courts to make a confiscation order in every case is onerous and unnecessary (cf Zander 1989). Others point out that, unless an investigation is made in every case, some traffickers who appear to have modest means but actually have substantial savings would emerge from prison (or, with minor offences, pay their fine), then to enjoy the proceeds of crime.

Escalation in imprisonment

The Misuse of Drugs Act 1971 increased the maximum penalties for what was then called drugs supply from ten to fourteen years for drugs such as heroin or cocaine. Subsequently, the Controlled Drugs (Penalties) Act 1985 increased the maximum penalty to life imprisonment.

Although the legislation does not prescribe minimum penalties, case-law from the Appeal Court has established a 'tariff' of imprisonment based on the supposed retail value of the drugs seized or presumed by the court to have been involved over a continuing period. These guidelines have an effect broadly similar to minimum penalties. Regarding the *supply* of heroin, the Lord Chief Justice, Lord Lane, thought that sentences would generally lie between three years and life: 'The sentence will largely depend on the degree of involvement, the amount of trafficking and the value of the drugs being handled' (Fortson 1988: 247). As regards *importation*, Lord Lane said, 'It is not difficult to understand why in some parts of the world, traffickers in heroin in any substantial quantity were sentenced to death and executed' (*ibid.*: 246). However, since this means of disposal is not available in Britain, a lesser scale of punishments was devised.

From the late 1980s onwards, trafficking a kilo of drugs such as heroin or cocaine (categorised as Class A, or most dangerous, under the Misuse of Drugs Act 1971) generally attracted a sentence of around ten years. Several such consignments or larger ones attracted a sentence of the order of fourteen years upwards. A few kilos of amphetamine (categorised as a medium-danger Class B drug) might attract a sentence around five years.

It is worth looking in some detail at the way the tariff is applied, since the implications for prospective traffickers are particularly clear. The basis of sentencing is

1 an appraisal by the court of the estimated money value (more properly, retail or street-level prices) of the consignment(s) of drugs
2 in some cases, especially those resting on conspiracy charges, the value taken for the purposes of sentencing will not be limited to the amount of drugs seized, but will be extended to include an amount value reckoned by the court to have been trafficked over an extended period
3 whether it appears that defendants genuinely believe (have good reason for believing) that they are handling a less dangerous drug
4 whether defendants plead guilty (in which case the sentence is reduced)
5 whether defendants are 'cooperative' in the sense that they name their contacts.[32]

From judgments handed down by the courts in Britain it appears that a combination of a guilty plea and giving information on other traffickers may result in a reduction in sentence by about one-third.

In a landmark case, for example, a sentence of twelve years was reduced to eight on appeal on just such grounds (*R* v. *Bilinski*, *Criminal Law Review* 1987: 783).

Whether the defendant is considered to be an organiser, likely to benefit considerably in financial terms, or simply a courier or 'mule', unlikely to see more than a tiny fraction of the consignment's selling price, is not a major consideration in sentencing. As Jane Goodsir, director of the legal advice agency Release, has noted, 'There's not much discrimination between the sentences on simple couriers and major dealers' (Bowcott 1990b: 6; see also Carvel 1990). In spite of the keenness to catch 'big traffickers' in the organisational sense, the courts have been unable to base punishment very much upon criteria of organisational size or market dominance. If the courts were to base punishment upon such criteria, then the likely result would be to impose much lower penalties on the run-of-the-mill traffickers who get caught. However, the relatively simple sentencing guideline of weight of drugs has come into use.

As regards the money value of the consignment, one practice in calculating this is to multiply the presumed or known wholesale-level price (e.g. price for amounts of a proportion of a kilo upwards) by a factor of between three and five, and to call the result the retail value. Sometimes a more complicated approach is followed, involving a series of assumptions about the purity of the drugs (which may vary throughout a consignment), the typical weight at which the drug would be sold to users, the typical purity at customer level, and the price customers pay to their immediate suppliers. Then, the total value of the consignment is calculated as follows (Kay 1988: 815).

Consignment weight × Consignment purity × Unit cost to customer

---

Typical unit weight at customer level × Typical purity at customer level

The assumptions made about each of these variables evidently affect the estimated consignment price. Indeed, when terms in such an equation are multiplied together, relatively small changes in the assumptions made can result in quite big changes in estimated consignment 'value'. It has been shown, for example, that a kilo of heroin in Britain 'could quite easily be calculated as worth £75,000, £300,000 or £900,000' (*ibid.*: 815). The potential consequences for offenders are considerable, since length of imprisonment is related to estimated consignment value.

However, the relationship between the value of drugs such as heroin or cocaine smuggled and the prison sentence likely to be imposed is not a linear one in Britain (Harvey and Pease 1987). The judgment of the Appeal Court in the case of *Aramah* (*Criminal Law Review* 1983:271–3) laid down guidelines at a time when the maximum sentence was fourteen years. These guidelines were subsequently amended in the case of *Bilinski* in the light of the increase in maximum penalty to life imprisonment. (Fortson 1988: 246; Bucknall and Ghodse 1989).

Estimated 'value' of drugs		*Sentence in years*
	Aramah (1983)	*Bilinski* (1987 onwards)
£1 million (many kilos)	12–14 years	14 years minimum
£100,000 (e.g. a few kilos of heroin)	7 years minimum	10 years minimum
An 'appreciable' amount (fraction of a kilo)	4 years	(no change specified)[33]

In other words, the risk–reward ratio *decreases* as one moves to larger consignments. People who are found guilty of trafficking in fractions of a kilo (say fifty grams or so, said to be worth around £5,000) are likely to get a sentence of the order of five years. This implies one year in prison for every £1,000 in retail value of the drug. But get caught with two kilogrammes – which might be worth around £100,000 at the retail level – and the sentence would be ten years and upwards. Here the tariff is one year for every £10,000 in retail value. The audacious trafficker, shifting many kilos worth say around £1.4 million, gets fourteen years minimum. Now the tariff is of the order of one-tenth of a year for every £10,000 worth in retail value. In other words, the prison sentence incurred for the tenth kilo is actually less than that incurred for the fifth kilo; the sentence for the fifth kilo is less than for the second, and so on.

Now, if there is any relationship between the pattern of crime and the system of controls in a society then the implications are fairly obvious. If one is going to traffick in heroin in Britain, then there is little point in restricting oneself to, let us say, one-quarter or half a kilo of heroin. The chances of being caught do not alter that much with increasing size of consignment (although they do with the number of consignments, due to the greater risks of a continuing operation). The implication for the calculating trafficker is rather similar to that old maxim, 'you might as well be hung for a sheep as a lamb'. One might as well traffick in as much as one can, in order to minimise the risk–reward ratio.

This is rather an odd set of inducements for a society supposedly concerned about trafficking.

THE ADMINISTRATION OF JUSTICE

Those caught face interrogation, committal for trial, remand in custody (in most cases), the court case, and sentencing, probable imprisonment and asset confiscation. In this section we examine some cases as they are processed through the criminal justice system.

We introduce the discussion of the disposal of prisoners by considering the question of remand – the power of the courts to order that persons accused be held in custody in the period up to their trial. The question of whether or not to remand a defendant in custody is quite often an issue between defence and prosecution. The defence, obviously, argues against remand, not only because being in prison for six months or so whilst the case come to trial is an unpleasant experience and can break up families and ruin careers, but also because it makes preparation of a defence more difficult.

The prosecution generally argues for defendants to be remanded in all but the more minor trafficking cases, either because of the danger of potential witnesses being intimidated or simply because defendants may flee. This outcome can be illustrated by completing the story of the Morgans, the firm of diversifiers described in Chapters 3 and 6. The case also illustrates the way in which a carefully constructed case can fail because the prosecution themselves feel obliged to withhold some evidence. The overall result is then hardly a victory for the police.

Two that got away

In the case of the Morgans the three men charged had been granted bail against sureties of £10,000 each. By the time the case reached court, one of the threesome (given the name Garry in Chapter 6) had left the country and, rumour had it, was in Spain. We

watched in court as one of the sureties, a local man, was called
to the witness stand by the trial judge. As the judge remarked, 'It
would appear on the face of it that you have stood surety in the sum
of £10,000 and that surety is in peril. I strongly advise you to take
legal advice.' The surety, presenting himself as a man let down by
others, claimed that it was actually another person who had stood
surety, and that he himself was simply a go-between who had
helped to arrange things by telephone. Be that as it may, the score
was now one defendant escaped, two to stand trial. Proceedings
were adjourned whilst enquiries were made, but the missing party
remained missing.

The re-convened trial then proceeded quite smoothly for the
prosecution, whose star witness was the undercover officer we
called Trevor in Chapter 6, who had set up this buy bust operation.
However, the prosecution laboured under difficulties related to
identification evidence. The second defendant, Colin, was arrested
some weeks after the arrest of the other two men. His role had been
to drive the car which contained the drugs and leave it in the car
park before departing the scene. In court his defence enquired as
to how the police could be sure of his identity having seen him
only briefly. The police had to admit that he had been arrested
later after being recognised by the undercover officer as someone
he had met several years ago. Pressed in court, Trevor said 'I
have met him on three previous occasions, with a person I've
been drinking with, but if I went any further it would reveal
my identity'. This is an odd expression to use whilst standing in
open court before the accused, and it may be that Trevor was
seeking to protect an informant who may have been present at
the same time. Protecting the identities of undercover officers
and of informants is a common issue in such cases (see Chapter
8).

This difficulty would have been overcome if the police had taken
a photograph of the person who escaped the scene of arrest.
Unaccountably, they had not. 'A balls up', according to one officer.
Another officer on surveillance duty at the scene also identified
Colin as having been there but, pressed by the defence, admitted
that he had previously been shown a photograph of the defendant.
Why did the police have a photograph of this defendant? Because
they had previous dealings with him. But what would the jury make
of that – would it not prejudice them against that defendant? The
judge declared

My reaction is one of great alarm and there is a danger of a grave miscarriage of justice. I do not believe that any direction from me . . . can possibly stop the jury coming to a conclusion based on speculation. I have come to the conclusion that the identification evidence ought not to be admitted.

Without admissible identification evidence, the case against Colin became untenable, and the judge ordered the jury to return a not guilty verdict. The score was then two free, one still on trial.

This left Dave, the third and last alleged member of the alleged gang. He was regarded by the police as a relatively minor member of the firm, but had been caught with the drugs in his car. Found guilty by the jury, he was sentenced to two years' imprisonment and ordered to pay £1,000 under an asset confiscation order.

From the point of view of the police, this result was rather disappointing, but better than nothing. It is, after all, an aspect of professionalism to be able to learn from one's mistakes, and try to do better next time.

Case study: from local bar to foreign cell

One of the by-products of the anti-trafficker push of the 1980s has been the number of women caught up in the drug enforcement effort (Carvel 1990). For some of those who have scraped by in the irregular economy for many years, the chance to make a few thousand pounds through acting as a courier or 'mule' can be hard to resist. Most of the non-British nationals in women's prisons are there for this reason (Women in Prison, personal communication). Roxanne's case provides an example, exemplifying the way in which officers try to 'work up the chain' from couriers to those who sent them.

Roxanne was born in the Unites States, is married and her husband is in prison. She has two children but is not eligible for welfare. She has no means of self-support. Whilst hanging around in a bar waiting for some prospect to turn up, Roxanne was approached by a man who bought drinks and then food, sounding her out about her circumstances. After meeting her on a second occasion, he suggested that she act as a courier, carrying cocaine from New York to Gatwick. She agreed. On arrival at Gatwick airport, she was stopped by a female officer who 'asked if I was carrying any drugs and first I said "no" but then I caught their eye and said "yes", because I knew I would be strip searched'.

In interrogation, after some prevarication, she described to Customs the man who sent her to Britain.

> I met him in a bar and we got into conversation. After four to six months he offered the job . . . I was supposed to get $7,000 and he gave me $2,300 and said the rest would be paid when I got back to the States. I have a strange feeling that the drugs were already paid for because everything happened so quick and he was so sure. I was supposed to take the Victoria line to Paddington [*sic*] and to phone a telephone number and to say that I was in a hotel which I was to choose and call the female and wait till she picked me up. Customs asked me if I was prepared to go through with this but I was afraid for my children so I did not. So then I was interrogated from 3.30 p.m. to about 1.00 a.m. in the morning.
>
> On the second visit of the Customs man I was shown photographs of a number of men and I recognised the Colombian who sent me. I went to court on a Monday and was sent for remand for three and a half months in Holloway. Legal aid was the only thing because I could not afford anything else, so I had [lawyers] Mr X and a Mr Y. At one point I said, 'do you think it would be wise to cooperate?' and he said, 'you know the saying, you scratch my back and I'll scratch yours'. Then they also said that it would be dangerous, and left it up to me. I basically saw the barrister once in the whole case. I said I want this over and done with.

> (Roxanne)

In court

> I pleaded guilty and I did cooperate to some extent with the Customs and a couple of weeks ago the person who sent me was arrested in this country. I got six years and I think that I got a high sentence and that they should have given me less than six. Before I got sentenced he [the Customs officer] said 'I'll help you reduce your sentence'. I asked Mr X [a solicitor], 'if I cooperate then what will I get?' and they said five years. On another occasion they said five to eight years.

Her information brought her 'employer' to court and she agreed to testify against him.

The guy from Customs said, 'I can help you and I can put in a good word for your first parole'. The questions I asked him were if I was going to get help with a deportation [i.e. immediate, not after parole release] and have a reduced sentence which I could serve in the United States. But I got no answers.

Roxanne says that Customs were consistently encouraging but unspecific.

The Customs man said that 'things can be solved – I have good news for you – your Colombian friend has been arrested and we need you to go in the witness box so that we can get the credit'. I said, 'but you have no answers for me' [on deportation] and he was going to see somebody at the Home Office, fine, but would he be honest enough? He needs me, he's been after this man for years.

A straightforward response would have been that the chances of immediate deportation were virtually nil. But such information would not have encouraged this woman in her belief that further cooperation would shortly re-unite her with her children. For convicted drug traffickers whom the enforcement agencies believe may be useful in trapping other traffickers, firm and binding agreements are certainly not the order of the day.

In such circumstances, offenders become worried that they may be putting themselves, family or friends at risk and yet may not get much in return.

I'm gonna be worried, I am worried because I'm going to be going into the witness box. I'm doing it because I've visualised things differently and I want my conscience clear and to feel that I did my share in correcting the error that I did and, anyway, I need to get out of here to see my children. I hope that they at least deport me. . . . They should know that I am not lying. I noticed that I was being used and he said, 'Help us to get somebody else', but I was involved in this one case, not anything else.

(Roxanne)

The case illustrates the emotional bargaining power that Customs have with some offenders, and also the practical limitations to that bargaining power in the absence of the authority to secure deportation for foreign nationals.

Case study: one who is angry

From the perspective of an outsider, Britain can seem 'a very barbaric country', in which the quality of justice available to foreigners is poor.

Carmen, a middle-class Colombian and a lawyer with her own legal firm, is serving a ten-year sentence for importation of cocaine. She maintains her innocence and has amassed documentary evidence which, she says, supports her theory of a 'fit-up' in Bogotá. Our interest here, however, will not be upon the question of guilt or innocence (this having been decided by the courts), but upon the *process* of being brought to trial and her subsequent attempts to appeal.

The case also raises a general point about the integrity of persons working for solicitors – Carmen has made a serious complaint against one solicitor. The firm and its employees may have behaved in an exemplary way, but there is undeniably scope for the kind of impropriety alleged.

Overall, the case illustrates the difficulties of conducting a defence when one does not speak the language of the country, when English classes are not available before one is convicted, when legal aid solicitors have limited resources and when one is of a 'suspect' nationality (in this case, Colombian).

The facts of the case are that Carmen, while visiting Britain together with another woman, and the latter's daughter, was arrested at Heathrow airport with just under a kilo of cocaine sewn into leather goods, transported in her baggage. Her baggage was delayed for some time, and when it eventually turned up she was challenged by a Customs officer who suggested that it was not her case. She, however, insisted that it was, and the three left the terminal and got into a taxi. Carmen was then detained by Customs and confronted with the cocaine. A legal aid solicitor, Mr First Solicitor, was called and Carmen was charged with importation. Her two travelling companions were questioned, no record was made of these interviews, and they were then released. First Solicitor and Co then represented Carmen at committal and at trial, mainly through the firm's Assistant Solicitor, who visited Carmen twice. She was remanded in police cells for three months, where she developed scabies from the dirty conditions. She was then moved to a prison and committed for trial.

At her trial, Carmen pleaded not guilty. The next day the jury retired but was unable to reach a verdict and so the judge ordered a re-trial. Why was the jury unable to agree a verdict in the first trial? In summary, the evidence was as follows.

Prosecution

Carmen was found to be importing cocaine, sewn into leather goods. She did not deny the goods were hers. She might well be a solicitor, but this in itself was not a guarantee against wrongdoing. True, she had been able to show that she was not poor since she had personal wealth in Colombia, but who was to say that this wealth was not the proceeds of past trafficking?

Defence

That there was cocaine in the leather goods was not disputed, but Carmen did not know it was there. She had been given the goods some weeks before her flight to London. Her explanation was that this man, whose amorous advances she had earlier refused, conspired with another man, whom she had sued for non-payment of a debt, to get her out of the way. The importation was not done 'knowingly' as required for a conviction.

Re-trial

At the second trial, the jury returned a guilty verdict after retiring for just over two hours. The judge handed down a sentence of ten years, based on the estimate that the 0.982 kilos of cocaine had a street value of £186,000. He also ordered a Confiscation Order under the Drug Trafficking Offences Act 1986, for £4,215 or 6 months' imprisonment in default, and recommended her for deportation at the end of her sentence. Since the sentence is over five years she is not likely to be paroled and will therefore serve at least six years.

Carmen has consistently maintained her innocence. She says that her older travelling companion was her client and had asked her to arrange an English course for her daughter. This she had done by telephoning a university in England and being advised by a Spanish-speaking member of staff that a local Academy would be suitable. She contacted the Academy, which sent her some literature. Carmen then accompanied Mrs Client and her daughter to England because Mrs Client is 'someone who can never travel. She has no experience of travel outside a small place. And she is a person who is very nervous, too much nervous, and she needs somebody to escort her when she travels.' However, she did not have any documentary evidence of this reason for her travel when she went to court.

As a solicitor herself, Carmen makes numerous criticisms of British law, of the conduct of her case, of the conditions of her imprisonment (e.g. police cells; of putting non-dangerous cases such as herself in high-security prison; of lack of language tuition therein), and of solicitors and the barrister acting for her. Her case certainly illustrates that being unable to speak the language, and being moved around the country, makes the organisation of a defence or an appeal very difficult. As she put it

> England is a very barbaric country to treat foreigners this way. The police talk very fast, your solicitors tell you to keep quiet, so you never get to exercise your defence. Then without proper instructions with barristers, you are just left feeling like a beauty queen, smiling and laughing, you don't know what is going on. This is the same for the Colombians, the Nigerians and the other Africans. My barrister said 'don't worry, it will be OK, it will be all right'.

Carmen's barrister observed in a memo to the solicitors that Carmen had been advised that sentence would be higher if she was found guilty after pleading not guilty, than if she pleaded guilty. The barrister also observed that the Court of Appeal in the case of *Bilinski* laid down a sentencing tariff of ten years and upwards for importation of Class A drugs with a street value of £100,000. The barrister advised that there were no grounds for appealing either verdict or sentence and said that legal aid would not be granted for any appeal.

Carmen has changed her solicitors several times. She first attempted to do so after Mr First Solicitor said that he had been suffering from illness and handed the case to his assistant. In 1989 Carmen made a complaint about this firm to the Solicitors Complaints Bureau, alleging that they inadequately prepared her case and that they failed to field the student as a witness at the trial. According to First Solicitor and Co, the student told them that she could not recall why Carmen was travelling with her and her mother. In direct contradiction, Carmen maintains that it was her legal advisers who recommended against calling this witness since she was another Colombian and hence unlikely to impress the Court. She says that she has a letter from the student offering to give evidence. The Solicitors Complaints Bureau, in a letter to Carmen, presented the situation as the student's unwillingness to give evidence. The Bureau also found that First Solicitor and Co did get evidence of Carmen's background and professional standing and presented it at the trial, and that there they could not be criticised on grounds of negligence.

After her sentence, Carmen was initially placed in Holloway Prison. She dismissed First Solicitor and Co and engaged the well-known London firm of Bad Reputation and Co and, at the same time (but against the advice she had been given by her barrister) initiated her own Leave to Appeal. Bad Reputation and Co's Mr Clerk (who subsequently left the firm and proved difficult to contact) attended her in Holloway to advise her about her appeal.

According to Carmen, she gave Bad Reputation's representative funds to pursue the appeal as a paying client. She has made allegations that, in the period leading up to the Leave to Appeal hearing, Bad Reputation's Mr Clerk took £2,000 or $2,000 for this purpose. Bad Reputation deny this, saying that only $250 was involved.

> [Mr Clerk] said to me, 'you have to pay me to start to work because I have to pay a barrister for advice and to pay for the work I have to do to go to court and do many papers for you. . . . Well, for a start, you can give me £2,000 and later when we get permission for the appeal maybe you can pay more'. And I asked him, 'how much more?' And he said 'well about three to four thousand pounds more'. Because I was very desperate, because of the situation, I said, 'well, I will ring my family and get the money'.

She says that she gave Mr Clerk $250 cash that day, getting this from her money held by the prison authorities. An equivalent sterling amount is recorded in Bad Reputation's books, and there is no conflict on this point. However:

> They gave me no receipt, nothing.
> Q. Did you ask for a receipt?

No, because I was very confused, I was in shock, I was very desperate.

She further claims to have given Mr Clerk another $400 cash at a second meeting, this money having been sent to her by her parents in the pockets of some clothes. Not having been found by the prison authorities, this amount was never held by them so there is obviously no record of it being passed over. Additionally, her family claims to have sent $1,500 cash by special delivery to Mr Clerk at Bad Reputation's. Neither of these two latter sums, $400 and $1,500, are recorded as having been received by Bad Reputation's.

Carmen pressed her complaint against Bad Reputation and Co. They put a denial in writing and said that only $250 had changed hands. Carmen was advised to 'get your family to send us at least £1,000 sterling' so that they could continue to represent her. Carmen complained to the Solicitors Complaints Bureau who replied that according to Mr Clerk and Bad Reputation's records, only $250 changed hands. No one asked about a receipt.

Clearly there is conflict of evidence here, between Carmen's version of events and Bad Reputation's. The firm and the individual may be quite blameless, but it is striking that by 1990 this particular firm had such a bad reputation amongst inmates and prison officers that little new business was coming their way from women prisoners.

Her first Leave to Appeal (against both verdict and sentence) before a single judge was rejected, the judge saying 'The jury heard your explanation and did not believe it. . . . Ten years for this offence upon a plea of not guilty and bearing in mind the amount and the value of the drugs is not excessive'. Mr Clerk then again visited her in prison and, she claims, talked about helping her with the next step of appeal, to the full Appeal Court.

And he said, 'yes, I know that [the first appeal was turned down], I've been in the court, but don't worry. We will now make the application for the full court, don't worry, it will work in the full court'. So he *with his own hand* [her emphasis] wrote in front of me the application for the full court. I have it here.

That was the last time she saw him. A few months later, her second Leave to Appeal was heard by the Appeal Court, and rejected. She was not represented at this hearing, indeed a person in Bad

Reputation's office appeared not to have been aware that Leave had been sought. This person, who later took over the case, wrote to Carmen saying that 'I have been trying to find out about your case but am having some problems contacting Mr Clerk'.

Around the time of her unsuccessful Leave to Appeal, Carmen was transferred to a high-security prison in the north of England, so she attempted to engage a more local firm of solicitors, Solicitor Number Three. She was seen by a partner of this firm. However, Carmen remained with Bad Reputation for a while, since in 1989 she was transferred to another prison which is nearer London. Following the failure of her complaint against Bad Reputation and Co, Carmen discharged that company and appointed Solicitor Number Four. However, she became dissatisfied with them when they asked to be put in funds to the tune of £1,000. She then attempted to change to Solicitor Number Five, a name suggested by the Colombian Consulate.

Carmen's experience of being processed through the criminal justice system is one that is shared in its essentials by many others. Had her case come to court in the early 1990s, when bilateral agreements would be in place between Britain and Colombia to allow the British courts to seize assets in Colombia, then her home and business would have been at risk as well.

WHAT ARE PENALTIES FOR?

What kinds of punishments, and at what levels, are in the public interest in relation to drug trafficking?

For some observers, the upwards escalation in penalties over the past two decades has been welcome, but the scale of the problem necessitates greater efforts. These further measures are merited not simply as a response to or deterrent against any involvement with drugs trafficking and consumption, but because of what that involvement is said to represent. For former US 'Drug Czar', William Bennett

> The drug crisis is a crisis of authority – in every sense of the term 'authority' . . . What can be done to combat this crisis of authority? Two words sum up my entire approach: consequences and confrontation. Those who use, sell and traffick in drugs must be confronted, and they must suffer the consequences. By consequences, I mean that those who transgress must make

amends for their transgressions. Consequences come in many forms. In terms of law enforcement, they include policies such as seizure of assets, stiffer prison sentences, revocation of bail rights, and the death penalty for drug kingpins. On these points I find general agreement. . . .

We need to do more. We need to reconstitute authority. What those of us in Washington, in the states, and in the localities can do is to exert the political authority necessary to make a sustained commitment to the drug war. We must build more prisons. There must be more jails.

(Bennett 1989: 4)

Such pronouncements rather exaggerate the degree of consensus that there is on matters of punishment. Not all Americans, for example, favour the death penalty and, in all probability, fewer Europeans would enthuse about it. Throughout the post-war years, penalties for trafficking have soared in virtually every country of the world, yet the problem remains. Is the death penalty the answer? Are more jails? Or imprisoning more people for longer terms?

A historical anomaly

In our view, the practical merits of long prison sentences for drug trafficking have not been established. Their preventive value has not been established. They are expensive to administer. Why then have such penalties?

Part of the answer is that these are expressive penalties, having as much or more to do with the declaration of disapproval of certain acts than with any real belief that they ameliorate the drug problem. Although in Europe there is less of a sense of the need to reconstitute authority than in the United States, that desire is certainly around. It has been in those terms of symbolic confrontation through enforcement that legislation and case-law on trafficking penalties have matured.

Although prison penalties (and traffickers' counter-measures) did go up considerably in the 1970s, the mid-1980s were the time of most rapid and publicised escalation. As Grieve notes,

Calls for the death penalty were met with the introduction of life imprisonment (Controlled Drugs Penalties Act, 1985). More severe sentences for drug trafficking alone went up from 12

years to 28 years in a four year period at the Central Criminal
Court.

(Grieve 1987: 163)

A massive escalation of imprisonment came to be perceived as
a modest reaction – perhaps even an under-reaction, by those
who favoured the ultimate sanction. Life imprisonment, in this
context, presented itself as the least that society could do. Even in
countries where there has been a sustained and relatively successful
attempt to reduce the average prison sentence, for instance The
Netherlands, prison terms for trafficking have bucked the general
trend, going up whilst most other sentences have gone down
(Downes 1988).

The escalation in the use of imprisonment for drug trafficking
runs counter to the general trend in the twentieth century for
the relative decline in the use of custody. As we indicated
above, financial penalties and various forms of punishment in
the community have tended to *replace* custody. In the case of
trafficking, however, there has been a doubling up process at work:
traffickers are nowadays much more likely to be imprisoned for a
long time if caught, *and* they are subject to financial penalties that
go beyond the concept of the fine to include asset confiscation.

It is time to look more closely at this anomaly. A fundamental
question is being overlooked. Do exceptionally long sentences do
any good, in the simple sense of restraining the drug market? This is
not an abstract question of whether imprisonment up to life ought,
according to some moral calculus of deterrence, to be of benefit.
Rather, it is a specific question: have escalating penalties over the
past few decades actually achieved their declared intention?

It has to be acknowledged that the rapid development of the scale
and sophistication of drug enforcement does have its successes, with
more and more people apprehended and convicted for a trafficking
offence, whereupon they serve long prison sentences. Yet, in spite
of this, drug markets continue to expand internationally and
domestically in most countries: trafficking thrives, drug availability
increases, use of illicit drugs is buoyant, going through changes in
fashion in regard of the substances concerned but hardly crumpling
under the onslaught of enforcement.

In our view, the original intention of the Hodgson Committee
in Britain, to deploy asset confiscation as a partial alternative to
longer terms of imprisonment, was a good one. Unfortunately,

like many proposals for reform in the criminal justice system, what was intended as an alternative became an adjunct. The virtually simultaneous passage of the DTOA and the Controlled Drugs (Penalties) Act 1985, causing the penalty of asset confiscation to be introduced alongside a further escalation of maximum prison sentences, shows an excess of gung-ho sentiments (Clutterbuck 1990) over careful analysis.

Looked at most positively, the criminal justice systems could use asset confiscation orders alongside a reduction in long prison sentences. But this potential has not been realised in relation to trafficking offences.

Conclusion
A little knowledge . . .

In parts I, II and III of this book we described the variety of forms that drug trafficking can take, and some responses of the enforcement agencies as they attempt to engage traffickers at national, county/city and local levels. We pointed to some important issues around covert operations, intelligence and punishment.

The discussion has at times been quite detailed and specific and, in moving towards an ending (if not closure), we should take a step backwards in order to get a view of how our research may be taken up and used. The covert nature of crime in general, and of drug trafficking in particular, means that it cannot ever be grasped directly in any full sense. It follows that trafficking can be portrayed in a variety of ways, depending upon the techniques and interests of those accredited to speak on the subject: the enforcement agencies; media; politicians; and, sometimes, criminologists.

In the closing pages, we mention some of the ways in which particular characterisations of trafficking, including our own account, may serve some specific interests.

'Greatest peace-time threat' (or, give us more resources)

Evidently, the intensity of the threat posed by trafficking may be played up or played down.

Playing up the threat is generally in the interests of law enforcement agencies, especially when they face budgetary constraints (as US and British enforcement agencies increasingly did from the mid-1980s onwards). Following the expansion of resources made available to law enforcement in Britain following the election of a Conservative government in 1979, the police have been caught up in the expectations of government and of the public that they would be able to demonstrate a significant impact on levels of crime. This expectation has not generally been met and the police now find their budgets are being related to indicators of their performance, rather than increasing in response to a gut feeling that enforcement is a good thing.

On the face of it, the police need to demonstrate that they are winning the war on crime, and that should perhaps lead them to abstain from declaring trafficking and other serious crime to be out of control. But, as Woodiwiss has pointed out, the lack of success of enforcement agencies may at least in part be explained away by emphasising the magnitude of the threat that they face, whereupon routine and bureaucratic concerns such as performance indicators and cost-effectiveness may be swept aside by a mobilisation of almost patriotic sentiment (Woodiwiss 1988). This seemed to happen in Britain for a while.

> We believe, from all that we saw and heard, that as the American market becomes saturated the flood of hard drugs will cross the Atlantic. We fear that unless *immediate* and effective action is taken Britain and Europe stand to inherit the American drug problem in less than five years. We see this as the most serious peacetime threat to our national well-being.
>
> (Home Affairs Committee 1985: para 2)

Opinion within the British police oscillates between playing trafficking up as a threat and playing it down. Since the 1989 crack panic, an increasing number of senior officers can be heard to say that 'war' analogies are inappropriate in this and other areas of policing.[34] It remains to be seen which way the police will go on this in future.

'Organised crime' (or, let's centralise enforcement)

One of the starting points for this research was the question of whether the popular representation of the market, as a static triangle or pyramid with a few big 'mafia'-type organised gangs sitting at the top and controlling the market, could be regarded as accurate.

There has perhaps been a rather crude de-bunking element in our work, as our reading of the literature, interviews with traffickers, and discussion with enforcement personnel fell quite easily into place in respect of this question. Of course, individual traffickers and the small groups that typically make up trafficker enterprises are organised in the sense that they are pursuing strategies designed to make a profit and keep as clear of enforcement agencies as possible. But there is no person, no mafia, no cartel organising the market overall. Rather, a large number of small organisations operate fairly autonomously of each other in a manner that may be described as 'disorganised crime' (cf Reuter 1983).

However, a literal rebuttal of the myth of organised crime may miss an important issue. Terms such as organised crime are significant not just as descriptions of criminality but, rather more, as ways of legitimising particular aspects of law enforcement. If crime is described as *organised* on a regional, national or even international level, then it seems to follow that enforcement agencies should be organised accordingly (ACPO 1985; for another view, see Dorn *et al.* 1991).

In Britain, the myth of organised trafficking has served a purpose, insofar as it was a crucial consideration in creating a near-consensus within the Association of Chief Police Officers, the Home Office and politicians that some degree of centralisation of policing was needed (Home Affairs Committee 1989b; 1990). The formation of the National Drugs Intelligence Unit, its role in 'piloting' the broader National Criminal Intelligence Service, and the elevation of the intelligence centre over local operational teams (see Chapter 9) effectively bequeaths to Britain a national detective agency along the lines of America's FBI.

What need, then, for further presentations of the myths of the 'big trafficker'?

'A diverse and fluid market' (or, do more low-level intelligence)

We have presented a view of drug markets as fluid, being made up of many diverse trafficking enterprises that change their modus operandi over time. In presentations of work-in-progress to audiences made up of enforcement personnel, we have found that although there might sometimes be disagreement over certain details, the general picture we presented was considered unremarkable. As one officer said to us in 1988, 'tell us something we don't know'.

Now there are several ways in which such a response may be taken. At one level, we have taken it as a kind of confirmation of the facts – we seem to have got it more or less right. At another level, we have worried that we may be missing something big and that it may be in everybody's interests to keep quiet about it. (In police parlance, let us carry on making prats of ourselves.) We doubt this, since the range of our respondents and the diversity of their interests militates against such a 'conspiracy theory'.

We come, then, to the question of the practical utility or consequences of acceptance of the view that the markets are made up of many small-to-medium trafficking enterprises, operating under many different guises. It seems to us now that such a view fits well with current trends for 'down market' enforcement (described in Chapter 7) and for more central collation and analysis of locally generated and often low-grade intelligence (Chapter 9). The emphasis on down-market policing – or *demand reduction* as it is often called – was initially signalled by the United States in its 1989 national drug control strategy (Office of National Drug Control Policy 1989) and subsequently endorsed by other countries at the April 1990 World Ministerial Summit to Reduce the Demand for Drugs and to Combat the Cocaine Threat.

It was only in the closing stages of our research that we began to set these trends alongside the centralisation and full computerisation of criminal intelligence in Britain, and the increasing use of undercover operations to 'develop' intelligence for possible future use. One of the implications is more effective surveillance of greater numbers of people, their movements, contacts, activities, financial affairs and so on (Foucault 1977; Marx 1988). This is probably not what most citizens have in mind when they think of drug enforcement – yet it is increasingly its emphasis, and one which we may have unintentionally given some support by our 'de-bunking' the big trafficker mythology.

'Clever and flexible traffickers' (or, please keep quiet about enforcement strategies)

It is a commonplace observation that criminals are keen students of the development of enforcement strategies, with an eye to developing effective counter-strategies. (See for example the account of anti-surveillance work by traffickers in Chapter 6.)

It is therefore not surprising that one oft-expressed concern about our own research was that it might betray current operational methods and act as a 'crime primer' which criminals might consult and adjust their operations accordingly. It was partly for this reason that we have relatively incomplete information on sell operations (Chapter 8). This is an understandable and legitimate concern for law enforcement agencies and one that to some degree squares with the wider public interest.

But there is a down-side to this, insofar as the need to keep criminals in the dark extends to a policy of keeping the public, and political representatives, equally in the dark. By stressing the flexibility of criminals, do we by implication and without intention lend support to the case for keeping quiet about the strategies and direction of law enforcement? Does not our research threaten to shade into support for the proposition that enforcement agencies must operate without accountability?

It seems important to us, therefore, to lay equal stress on the flexibility and creativity of the enforcement agencies so that, even if their modus operandi yesterday are known, it can be argued that this gives little away to criminals about what is likely to be the case today or tomorrow. We are left, however, with the conundrum that a basic social science perspective on traffickers – as open to learning in their interactions with enforcement agencies within the wider social environment – tends to translate into an argument for greater secrecy and non-accountability of enforcement agencies.

In closing, let us observe that the pursuit of *truth* about drug trafficking is one way of thinking, whilst the question of the *purposes served* by any particular grasp on the truth may be just as important. The ambitions of this study have primarily run along the first line of thought but, as our copy date approached, we became more perplexed by the second. Would we do it all again in the same manner? We might or, there again, we might not. Like traffickers, enforcement agents and readers of books, social scientists are capable of learning and change.

Appendix

Extracts from ACPO's Broome Report

INTRODUCTION: A WAY-STATION IN THE REORGANISATION OF POLICING

Britain, unlike most other developed countries, has no national detective agency. The reasons for this are historical and quasi-constitutional, local police forces being formally accountable (in other than 'operational' matters) to local Police Committees of their city or county. Only the Metropolitan (London) Police are answerable to the Home Secretary, and successive Home Secretaries have been reluctant to extend this control more widely since to do so would remove the 'partial autonomy' enjoyed by the police and risk allegations of direct political control.

Nevertheless, there has been a historical tendency towards centralisation, with smaller police forces being amalgamated into larger ones; the development of Regional Drug Squads to combat serious crime; and the growth of a National Criminal Intelligence Service, based in part on the model of the National Drugs Intelligence Unit (previously the Central Drugs Intelligence Unit of the Metropolitan Police, from the days when drugs were seen as a London concern).

As described in Part III of this book, and in Chapter 9 in particular, it was mainly through the extension and reorganisation of the intelligence function of policing that this centralising tendency has shown itself in recent years. Intelligence is shifting from being a subsidiary aspect of policing to being its active centre. It now has a much more directive role – that of 'intelligence development' – which, it is anticipated, will increasingly involve centrally generated directives to local and regional forces.

Thus, it is through the development of criminal intelligence in general, and drugs intelligence specifically, that Britain is seeing movement towards a *de facto* national detective agency. As one senior officer rather gloomily expressed the manner of this movement, it seems the British way to inch oneself along, bit by bit, rather than declaring one's target and pledging oneself to attain it. Alongside this reticence, however, we must acknowledge the existence of differences of opinion in the police service about how far the trend to centralisation should go, and a degree of sensitivity over how it might be perceived politically.

The Association of Chief Police Officers has kindly allowed us to reproduce extracts from its 1985 Working Party on Drugs Related Crime (the 'Broome Report', so called after its chair, then Chief Constable of Avon and Somerset). Although the question of organisation of detective policing was not explicitly included in the terms of reference (see below), this was very much on the agenda, as the introduction of the report makes clear. As paragraph 3 says, discussion at the preceding (1984) National Drugs Conference of ACPO 'largely centred around the idea of creating a regional or national police structure to tackle the drug problem'. After deliberation, the Working Party decided against recommending a national operational squad as such.

However, in a move that has turned out to be at least as significant as its recommendations on the regional level of drug enforcement, the Working Party made a number of recommendations about the organisation of drugs intelligence. In particular, it recommended the establishment of the National Drugs Intelligence Unit, which since 1988 has been under the auspices of Home Office Central Services. This may be regarded as a pilot or 'dry run' for the subsequent creation of the National Criminal Intelligence Service (operational in 1992). It also made recommendations that influenced the way in which British legislators took up the recommendations of the Hodgson Committee on asset confiscation (described in Chapter 10).

All in all, the Broome Report, as a historical document, provides an insight into the thinking of senior officers in Britain. This is of importance for all of us since, it seems to us, what ACPO decides today, we shall be debating tomorrow.

ASSOCIATION OF CHIEF POLICE OFFICERS
FINAL REPORT OF WORKING PARTY ON DRUGS
RELATED CRIME

Editorial note

In editing the report for publication here, we have deleted passages that seem to us to have little policy relevance or which present factual information now overtaken by the passage of time. The original paragraph numbers have been retained, so the reader can see where a deletion has occurred. The full report can be consulted in the reference library of the Institute for the Study of Drug Dependence, 1 Hatton Place, Hatton Garden, London EC1N 8ND; (library 071-430 1993).

INTRODUCTION

National Drugs Conference

3 Discussion at the 1984 National Drugs Conference largely centred around the idea of creating a regional or national police structure to tackle the drug problem. However it was apparent that to restrict the Working Party to that single facet would mean that possible improvements in other areas of police response would be overlooked. Equally whilst the police effort is diverse, its component parts are not mutually exclusive but are inter-related and interdependent.

Terms of reference

4 Broad terms of reference were necessary and they were drawn up and approved. They were:

As far as it relates to the Police Service in England and Wales:
(a) To consider and evaluate the nature and extent of the problem of unlawful activities connected with the production, manufacture, importation, distribution, purchase, sale and mis-use of drugs controlled by the criminal law, and the importance of drug-related offences in the broad context of crime;

(b) To review the effectiveness of the police action in the enforcement of the law connected with drugs offences; additionally to examine the co-operation which exists between the agencies involved in achieving common aims;

(c) To make recommendations on changes needed to improve present arrangements for the prevention and detection of such offences and for tackling the problems at Force, Regional and National levels, including any changes in training required. . . .

PART ONE – THE PROBLEM

Comment on the indicators

1.36 Whilst the increased scale of drug misuse has been identified, its changing nature has also been noted. No longer is the problem confined to the young or particular socio-economic groups. There is evidence that a geographical and societal distribution of drug abuse has occurred, with drugs appearing in semi-urban and rural areas, and amongst all groups in the community.

1.37 The involvement of organised criminals in the lucrative area of trafficking in drugs means that there is a greater sophistication in the importation and distribution process. The rewards are great and accordingly have attracted professional criminals who hitherto were involved in robbery and other serious crime. High profit and uncomplaining victims make the drug trade vulnerable to the involvement of professional criminals. A recent Metropolitan Police study revealed that 25 per cent of all target criminals were involved in drug activity of some kind. . . .

PART TWO – POLICE RESPONSE

H. M. Customs – responsibility

2.23 Historically H. M. Customs has assumed a responsibility for importation offences with the 43 Police Forces dealing with possession and supply offences and the illicit manufacture of drugs within the United Kingdom. This division of work continues to the present day.

Developing levels of response

2.24 Similarly over the past years a discernible pattern for tackling drug misuse at different operational levels began to be identified, i.e. Divisional, Force and Regional/National levels.

2.25 Clearly there are different levels of approach which match the different stages in the drug distribution process. The uniform officer will encounter simple possession offences with his Force Drug Squad colleague in the main dealing with small or medium level distributors. The major importer and distributor is now being increasingly targetted by Regional Crime Squads. These different approaches and varying stages in the drug distribution process are not distinct and at times they merge and overlap.

The three-tier approach

2.26 However, it is possible to formulate a strategy which should act as a series of checks against drugs misuse. First we must have a strategy of preventing importation and distribution and this must be done in conjunction with H. M. Customs. Secondly Force Drug Squads must tackle drug distribution where it has evaded the first level of control. Finally all officers at Divisional level should seek to remove drugs that reach street level. This approach should be identified and co-ordinated and it is necessary to examine this strategy in greater detail, together with the organisation and intelligence structures that are required to effect it.

PART THREE – ENFORCEMENT OPTIONS

Introduction

3.1 When examining the drug problem it became apparent to the Working Party that the effort against drug abuse can effectively be structured on three levels. In many respects this already occurs, but in our view a clear strategy needs to be identified. . . .

Divisional level

3.3 The lower tier should be based firmly at Divisional level. Uniform and Divisional detective officers are increasingly involved in drugs investigation. In the main their activity is centred on simple possession offences or small scale supply and in investigating crime which might be related to drugs, i.e. burglary, fraud, etc. . . .

Force level

3.5 At Force level Force Drug Squads are ideally placed to concentrate their activity against medium level dealers as well as co-ordinating Force intelligence on drugs. What is also required however is a clear definition of all their responsibilities at that level. . . .

Regional and national level

3.7 At regional or national level the Regional Crime Squads are involved in 'targetting' major distributors, who are often importers, often acting on information provided by the Central Drugs Intelligence Unit. Their activities have on occasions an international dimension and require liaison with other agencies, i.e. H. M. Customs, in cross-region or national investigations. . . . There is a need for a dedicated body of men working at this level.

Co-ordinated three-tiered approach

3.9 All officers within the three-tiered system should be briefed as to their own responsibilities and those of their Divisional, Force and Regional colleagues. The need for the gathering and evaluation of intelligence so crucial to drugs investigation must be underlined. . . .

3.14 . . . the sheer scale of the problem facing this country arising from drug abuse is so large that other alternatives must be examined. The efforts of H. M. Customs and police at regional/national level determines what proportion of drugs reaches street level. It is at the national level that our response has to be formidable and effective. It was with this in mind that the Working Party examined the various options in some detail.

National Drug Squad

3.15 One possible solution towards detecting large-scale importers and suppliers of controlled drugs is to consider the formation of a separate National Drug Squad for England and Wales. The proposal has been made in a number of quarters over recent years and is regarded by many, particularly those outside the Service, as being an attractive solution.

3.16 Given that importers and suppliers of drugs operate throughout the country without the constraint of city, county or regional boundaries, offenders can be said to operate in a national context. It follows therefore that a National Unit may be required to identify those offenders. Most of the successful operations against major offenders have required observations to be kept and enquiries to be made in many different parts of the country and have often required simultaneous searches and arrests in diverse parts of England and Wales. The geographical scope of police operations is determined by the extent of the criminal's operation and his need to import drugs either through air or sea ports or on some remote stretch of coastline or a landing strip. So it follows that if major importers and suppliers operate nationally then, the argument goes, police response should be nationally based.

3.17 Our present arrangements using Force Drug Squads and Regional Crime Squads can inhibit cross-Force or regional boundary enquiries. Often it is difficult to identify which Force or region holds the pre-eminent and therefore controlling position in the operation. Secondly it has to be said that on occasions the common good that can be derived from joint enquiries is affected by parochialism. . . .

3.19 A National Drug Squad staffed by officers from all constituent Forces in England and Wales financed and equipped on a per capita basis would not be inhibited by boundaries or parochial considerations.

3.20 A main office probably in London could have satellite offices in other provincial areas. Utilising national and international intelligence; it could target major importers and suppliers and concentrate solely on operations of national concern . . .

3.22 A direct relationship with the Central Drugs Intelligence Unit would be established with both organisations forming a twin-pronged intelligence/operational unit. . . .

3.25 As a blue print solution to the problem, a National Drug Squad is at the first instance a very attractive option. It would certainly co-ordinate and improve our existing regional and national effort and contains many of the required elements.

3.26 This solution has however one major disadvantage. Constitutionally it would be a new and radical innovation in British policing. There is considerable antipathy to the idea of a National Police Force. This would be seen by many as a step in that direction and would be likely to arouse strong opposition. In the current climate significant difficulties would be encountered if such a measure were to be favoured. However this in itself should not necessarily mean that the Service should reject this move. It is necessary to examine the constitutional implications a little closer.

3.27 We would have for the first time an operational commander of a national police unit and it is difficult to see how he could be answerable to local authorities as Chief Constables are. In effect the constitutional tripartite approach to policing would be broken.

3.28 Even if such an officer were to be made constitutionally responsible to an ACPO local or central authority, such responsibility could only be in the broadest terms and effectively firm operational control could not be exercised.

3.29 Certainly if he were to be made responsible to the Home Secretary there would be the innovation of Central Government having a direct operational responsibility for a police unit.

3.30 In effect the Unit would suffer forever the fundamental criticism that it is operating without effective restraint or constitutional supervision.

3.31 Similarly concern would be felt by many Chief Officers that a national police unit was operating within their areas and yet effectively outside their control. There are clearly significant implications to the operational autonomy and responsibility of Chief Constables for their own Force areas in the establishment of such a unit. . . .

3.33 A further flaw in the argument for a National Drug Squad is that in order to achieve the benefits of greater co-ordination and an effective police strategy at regional and national level, it is not necessary to go so far as to create a national unit. Whilst major drugs operations are geographically extensive, there are few examples of any major drug distributors operating on a truly national scale. What really happens is that there is a criminal conspiracy with tentacles of that conspiracy stretching to other areas but not throughout the entire country.

3.34 It could be argued that the constitutional opposition to such an idea has been already overcome by the establishment of the Regional Crime Squad and the post of National Co-ordinator of Regional Crime Squads. However they are essentially regionally based and answerable to a Regional Chief Constables Committee and the Regional Local Authority Committee for their operational and financial requirements respectively.

3.35 Any future drugs unit designed to deal with major drugs offenders needs mobility and the freedom to operate across Force boundaries; it does not require a national basis. In our opinion to enter into the constitutional difficulties previously mentioned is a questionable exercise and probably counter productive to the Service.

3.36 Additionally drugs related crime is interwoven with other crime. To isolate it and create a National Unit to tackle it may mean other officers would not see the problem as their responsibility. . . . The Working Party, after consideration of these issues, does not recommend the formation of a National Drug Squad. . . .

Regional Drug Squads

3.44 If constitutional and operational considerations pre-empt the formation of a National Drugs Unit or Task Force, then it is necessary to examine the concept of regionally based drug units.

3.45 In essence such units exist now in the form of the Regional Crime Squads. It is necessary however to examine in greater detail whether this system is adequate and effective or whether it requires strengthening in some way.

3.46 The Regional Crime Squads are successful in major drugs investigation. Their record speaks for itself. Their responsibilities are numerous, with considerable burdens being placed upon them whenever major crimes are committed. The Working Party are firmly of the view that Regional Crime Squads in their present form cannot absorb additional drugs work particularly if it is part of an overall co-ordinated strategy which in itself will precipitate additional tasks.

3.47 The extent to which the Regional Crime Squads are now involved in drug investigation work has been assessed and described in Appendix 'C'. They are slowly becoming

Regional Drug Units with consequent effects on their other responsibilities. Their workload and the fact that many Force Drug Squads cannot carry out major drug investigations has led to a report from the C.D.I.U. that some drugs intelligence is not being acted upon owing to lack of operational resources.

3.48 This development is now raising questions about whether this drift towards more involvement in drugs investigation can be allowed to continue. . . .

3.50 . . . formation of Regional Drug Squads has to be considered.

3.51 There are considerable attractions to the formation of [Regional Drug Squads]. They would be able to play a positive role in a co-ordinated tiered approach to drugs misuse. They would allow the Regional Crime Squad to adhere more closely to their traditional and vital policing role. They would be dedicated and tasked specifically towards one area of police activity and would quickly acquire expertise and experience in that field. Liaison with other agencies and the use of drugs intelligence would improve and C.D.I.U. would have a dedicated operational arm to whom they could direct their intelligence. Therefore on operational grounds and in recognition of the serious challenge posed by drugs, the Working Party came to the inevitable conclusion that some form of regional drugs investigation effort needed to be established. . . .

3.55 A further alternative is to establish Regional Drug Units and place them under the aegis of the Regional Crime Squads. They could assume responsibility for drugs investigation allowing their Regional Crime Squad colleagues to revert to their other responsibilities as defined in their terms of reference.

3.56 The Regional Crime Squads system is effective and already exists with a structure of administration, supervision and financial control answerable locally to a Chief Constables Management Committee, and nationally to a Standing Committee on Regional Crime Squads. In effect, an organisational structure exists within which such units could be located obviating the need for new supervisory ranks and other costly considerations.

3.57 In essence there are sound financial and organisational reasons for establishing dedicated Regional Drugs Units within the organisational umbrella of the Regional Crime Squad and it is so recommended.

Recommended new structure

3.58 The detail of such units needs to be examined. It is suggested that such units comprise one Detective Inspector, four Detective Sergeants and eight Detective Constables co-ordinated by a Detective Chief Inspector. It is suggested that the existing post of Detective Chief Inspector (Crime Intelligence) be utilised for this purpose. He would be answerable to the Regional Co-ordinator.

3.59 We believe that in accordance with the present Regional Crime Squad structure, the National Co-ordinator should act as the national focus for the efforts of the new Units. He would be responsible for reporting on a regular basis to a Standing Committee on Regional Crime Squads which should reflect the Regions by representation at Chief Constable level.

3.60 In its new role the constitution of the Standing Committee should be re-examined reflecting as it should a greater operational involvement and requiring a Chief Constable to chair it. This we see as essential to recognise the constitutional position of Chief Constables. . . .

Command structure

3.69 We have shown the necessity for a three-tier strategy towards drug investigation and have made recommendations as to how a regional/national effort should be organised, and later in the report make suggestions concerning intelligence. We recommended that the National Co-ordinator of Regional Crime Squads assume responsibility for co-ordinating such investigations. . . .

PART FOUR – DRUGS INTELLIGENCE

Introduction

4.1 Reliable intelligence is at the heart of all successful drug investigations. If a co-ordinated strategy against drugs is to be created then a similar approach as regards the obtaining, evaluation and dissemination of drug intelligence is required.

Present structure – Local level

4.2 At local level there is a well-established system of collators or local intelligence officers who obtain and disseminate local drug intelligence or pass on information having a wider relevance. The Working Party is satisfied that changes at that level are not required.

Regional level

4.3 At regional level there is the structure of Regional Criminal Intelligence Offices. Their role in drugs intelligence is small. R.C.I.O.'s have intelligence links with the Regional Crime Squad and because of 'targetting' some drugs intelligence becomes available to them. Again some contact exists between Regional Criminal Intelligence Offices and the Central Drugs Intelligence Unit but not in any formal structured way.

Central Drugs Intelligence Unit

4.4 Recommendations can be made regarding regional intelligence, but it is necessary first to examine closely the role of the Central Drugs Intelligence Unit. Created in 1972 it now fulfils different functions to those originally intended, but the Unit has proved effective.

4.5 The Working Party during its deliberations came to the view that the Unit is a success story and pay tribute to the forethought of its creators. Indeed if it had not existed this Working Party would have been recommending the creation of such an organisation.

4.6 A national drugs intelligence centre linked into the international network and staffed by officers from every police region of the United Kingdom, is an integral part of any police strategy against drug misuse.

4.7 Over the years deficiencies have been identified. One early criticism was that the Unit primarily received but did not transmit intelligence. This was largely due to the need for the Unit to 'sell' itself to Police Forces in the hope that they would 'trade' with it. Little time was spent on evaluating and disseminating intelligence. This has now changed with all Forces giving and receiving information and intelligence on a regular basis and the evaluation and dissemination of intelligence is now a major part of its overall effort.

4.8 Indeed as mentioned, the Unit is now in the position of having a surfeit of high quality intelligence. This surfeit revealed a dearth of operational capability to use it. Either Force Drug Squads have not the capacity to handle it or the Regional Crime Squads are fully occupied. This single fact of quality intelligence awaiting action underlines powerfully the need for a more structured response to drugs, and persuaded considerably the Working Party towards their recommendations on the formation of Regional Drug Units. . . .

PART FIVE – LIAISON WITH OTHER AGENCIES

National and regional consultation

5.31 Comment has been made from certain quarters that there are difficulties in dealing with 43 different Forces. The structure of ACPO, with its well established system of regional and national liaison, and its consultation with other agencies and organisations, has shown that the Police Service can approach matters from a regional or national perspective. The events of the past 12 months prove the truth of this. There appears to be no reason why H. M. Customs and the Police Service cannot display such an approach on the drugs issue.

PART SEVEN – SEIZURE OF ASSETS

Present powers of the courts

7.1 During our discussions we became aware of the vast profits to be made out of trafficking in drugs. It was apparent that no effort by the law enforcement agencies would be totally effective without the mechanism to take away such profits in order to prevent further financing of drug distribution networks. . . .

Tracing assets

7.7 What is needed is first of all an effective means of tracing assets. It is essential that police should be able to trace assets successfully both nationally and internationally or the whole concept of seizure of assets as a weapon against major drug dealers collapses. It is no good giving extra powers to the courts thereafter.

7.8 Tracing of assets in suitable cases should be done prior to a court appearance in parallel with the criminal investigation. We feel that there should be a power, available only on application by the Director of Public Prosecutions to a Judge of the High Court on proof of reasonable grounds for suspecting that a person is dealing in illicit drugs, for the police to inspect financial records of persons or organisations. Powers of search should be included. Such a financial investigation should be done by police officers with customs officers, accountants and Inland Revenue investigation officers as appropriate, and should run parallel to the main investigation incorporating restraint orders as necessary in order to freeze identified assets. This is not a new idea. The formation of such a procedure was recommended in the report of the Royal Commission on Standards of Conduct in Public Life when considering the prevention of corruption. In fact many of the excellent arguments put forward in that report apply equally well to drugs dealing – both being diseases that spread alarmingly if not dealt with by special measures.

7.9 Incorporated into the financial investigation should be the ability to obtain information held in confidence by the Inland Revenue and other official agencies. At a time when we are asking other countries to assist us by making provision for financial dealings to be disclosed, within this country the police are pro-hibited from finding out, for the common good, the financial assets of major drugs dealers. Once again the arguments put forward in the Royal Commission Report mentioned above are very persuasive. . . .

Reversal of the burden of proof

7.11 Having established that assets are in the ownership or under the control of a suspect, we see the next step involving the reversal of the burden of proof. There is resistance to this in principle in various quarters but we see it as an essential prerequisite of success.

7.12 There is a precedent in the Prevention of Corruption Act, 1916, which was introduced following comments made by a Trial Judge about the inadequacy of penalties for offences involving corruption in Government Wartime Contracts. Under that Act, where it is proved that a gift or consideration has been received by an employee of the Crown or any public body from a contractor, the onus lies on the defence to prove that the gift or consideration was not given or received corruptly. We see no reason why this principle which has existed for 69 years in the case of corruption, should not be extended to drugs dealing.

The Hodgson Report

7.13 The report of a Committee under the Chairmanship of Sir Derek HODGSON entitled 'The Profits of Crime and Their Recovery' has been considered by the Working Party. We feel that the recommendations in the report fall well short of what would be required to be effective against major drugs dealers. . . .

7.16 There must be a recognition that any person who involves himself in trafficking and dealing in drugs puts himself in jeopardy, not only from imprisonment following a criminal conviction (and here we applaud the recent Government announcement that the maximum term of imprisonment for drugs trafficking is to be increased), but also from a detailed fiscal examination and forfeiture of his financial assets. . . .

7.18 The recommendations may seem draconian but many of the suggestions are the same as procedures already existing in other Western countries. They are in our view well justified in view of the current serious drug problem.

7.19 However, it is acknowledged that there are difficulties in establishing and agreeing such sweeping legislative powers in the short term. . . .

Home Office proposals

7.20 In essence they revolve around pre-trial restraint, confiscation by means of fine, and compatibility with legislation implemented in other countries. They pay due regard to the complexities involved as for example confiscation of assets belonging to the offender's family and the need to ensure that previous transactions are 'for value'. The proposals to create an offence to acquire, possess, use or launder the proceeds of drug trafficking, together with the ability to impose considerable fines where assets are outside the jurisdiction of the courts, are also included.

7.21 We consider that these proposals are a useful first step towards establishing legislative provision for confiscation and forfeiture procedures. The creation of the offence of using the proceeds of drug trafficking is a very appealing option based as it is on a similar provision operative in Canada which has proved particularly useful.

7.22 However we do have reservations on the use of fines as a means of confiscating assets. Fines relate to punishment for an offence and reflect the financial status of the convicted person. They have a role in ensuring a just penalty but in our view are not always an appropriate way of confiscating assets other than those relating to a particular crime and the courts in our view may take this stance. Where assets cannot be effectively seized, for example if invested overseas, then there is a good case for a fine that reflects this. We do not feel that it will be effective to rely entirely on fines. Neither do we feel that the use of fines should, or would, obviate the need for very searching enquiries by the police into assets held. . . .

PART EIGHT – TRAINING

Introduction

8.1 Training should reflect the task of the person to be trained. This is nowhere more true than in the police effort against drugs misuse. For example, an officer working at the top level against major importers and distributors may require extensive training in surveillance, buying and other dangerous undercover work. At the lower level, officers on street patrol need to know, amongst other things, how local police policy integrates with the work of other local agencies. . . .

Additional training needs

8.6 Elsewhere in this report we have identified a three-tier approach which we feel is essential in our overall strategy. We suggest that there is a need for the different levels of approach at Divisional, Force, Regional and National level to be clearly reflected in training. It is acknowledged that it is not possible to draw up clear demarcation lines between the different levels and it is accepted that responsibilities will overlap. Nevertheless it is felt that a fairly clear assessment could be made of the relative responsibilities of each. . . .

8.8 At all levels officers' awareness of their roles in an overall police strategy will need to be underlined as well as their involvement with other agencies. . . .

PART ELEVEN – SUMMARY OF RECOMMENDATIONS

Part one – The problem	Paragraph	Page
1. That drug statistics on indicators be provided at an earlier time in order that effective resource decisions can be made.	1.45	12

Part three – Enforcement options

	Paragraph	Page
2. That police operational strategy be based on a three-tiered approach i.e. Divisional Force and Regional/National levels.	3.2	20
3. That increases in the strength and equipment of some Force Drug Squads are essential.	3.6	21
4. That all officers at each level of police response should have a clear, unambiguous appreciation of their particular responsibilities.	3.9	21
5. That Regional Crime Squads be augmented by a drugs wing under the supervision of a Detective Chief Inspector responsible to the Regional Co-ordinator and consisting of units of one Detective Inspector, four Detective Sergeants and eight Detective Constables.	3.57 3.58	31
6. That the existing post of Chief Inspector (Intelligence) of the Regional Crime Squad be utilised supervisor of the Regional Drugs Unit responsible to the Regional Co-ordinator.	3.58	31

7. That the National Co-ordinator of the   3.59   31
    Regional Crime Squads act as a national
    focus for the efforts of the Regional
    Drug Units, similar to his existing duties
    for Regional Crime Squads.

8. That the National Co-ordinator report to   3.59   31
    the Standing Committee on Regional
    Crime Squads on the work of Regional
    Drug Units.

9. That the Standing Committee on   3.60   31
    Regional Crime Squads should have
    regional Chief Constable representatives
    and be chaired by a Chief Constable.

10. That the disposition of Regional   3.63   32
    Drug Units as outlined at Appendix 'D'
    be adopted.

11. That when the Metropolitan Police   3.66   33
    complete the evaluation of their response
    to drugs abuse, that the need for a
    regional drug response in the No. 9
    Region be re-examined.

12. That the terms of reference of the   3.72   34
    National Co-ordinator of Regional Crime
    Squads be re-examined to take account of
    possible additional responsibilities.

13. That the rank of the National   3.73   34
    Co-ordinator be similarly examined.

14. That the Chairman of the body   3.74   34
    reviewing Regional Crime Squads be
    provided with a copy of this report.

Part four – Drugs intelligence

15. That the Central Drugs Intelligence   4.12   37
    Unit be renamed the National Drugs   4.13
    Intelligence Unit and be placed under
    the control of the National
    Co-ordinator of Regional Crime
    Squads.

16.	That the National Drugs Intelligence Unit continues to be responsible to the Steering Committee on the C.D.I.U. through the National Co-ordinator.	4.16	38
17.	That the National Drugs Intelligence Unit remains within New Scotland Yard.	4.16	38
18.	That either the Chief Superintendent or Superintendent (Deputy) of the National Drugs Intelligence Unit should always be a Metropolitan Police officer.	4.16	38
19.	That within England and Wales the structure of drugs intelligence be approached on three levels, i.e. Divisional, Force and Regional/National levels, commensurate with the three-tiered operational approach.	4.17	38
20.	That existing collator/local intelligence offices and Force intelligence systems are appropriate for evaluating and disseminating local and Force drugs intelligence.	4.18	38
21.	That Regional Criminal Intelligence Offices assume a responsibility for evaluating and disseminating regional drugs intelligence and for liaising with N.D.I.U.	4.24	39
22.	That N.D.I.U. field liaison officers be based within Regional Criminal Intelligence Offices in all Police regions of the United Kingdom.	4.28	40
23.	That there should be one data base for major drugs intelligence at the N.D.I.U. for use by police and H. M. Customs and that discussions to bring this into being should take place as soon as possible.	4.33	41
24.	That all international drugs intelligence be provided to the international desk of the N.D.I.U. by the police and H. M. Customs.	4.39	43

research initiative on the lines
described in this report.

32. That discussions with the Home Office   6.27   56
should take place to identify areas of
primary and other research likely to be
of assistance to law enforcement.

Part seven – Seizure of assets

33. That H. M. Government in its proposed
legislation to grant powers to courts
as regards 'asset stripping' should
take account of the following points:

    (a) That the ability to seize the   7.1   57
         profits derived from drug
         trafficking is an absolute
         necessity as a means of
         effectively controlling its
         spread;

    (b) That there should be a rebuttable   7.11 and   59
         presumption that in prescribed   App 'E'
         circumstances assets have been
         derived from drug trafficking and
         this presumption will operate for
         a period of ten years prior to the
         first offence date for which an
         offender is charged;

    (c) That the powers should allow a   7.16   60
         fiscal examination of an
         accused's assets.

Part eight – Training

34. That the ACPO Training Committee be   8.10   64
asked to re-examine the training
requirements of officers in relation to
drugs.

Part nine – The Forensic Science Service

Notes

1 A note on the use of the terms 'trafficking' and 'traffickers'. These words entered the British vocabulary on social problems in the 1980s, following north American usage. They were 'adopted' into legislation by the Drug Trafficking Offences Act 1986. For a discussion, see Chapter 10.

2 It is instructive to consider such amateurish infiltration and surveillance of the 1960s with the more rigorously conceived techniques and ploys of the 1980s, described in Chapter 6. The same over-the-top amateurism is displayed in Pritchard's account of his work as an undercover drug squad officer in the 1960s, see Pritchard and Laxton on 'The tricks of the trade', (1978: 28 and *passim*).

3 Such studies have provided rich portraits of criminal worlds, but we might also note the possible danger that too much of this kind of sympathetic or celebratory account of charismatic characters and sad failures (almost invariably white males) could do as much of a disservice to criminological ethnography as was done to youth culture studies by a similar body of masculine praise for the 'symbolic significance' of the rituals of young, white males in the 1970s.

4 Lyman (1987: 65) describes three functions which can be played by persons acting in a counter-surveillance capacity: an intelligence team would be informing on the presence of law enforcement people in the vicinity; tactical team 1 would entail acting as an armed body guard to prevent 'rip-offs'; and tactical team 2 would be to aid the dealer in escaping from police arrest.

5 In Lyman's (1987: 65) terms, the 'joeys' are performing a counter-surveillance function (cf note 4 above).

6 The name of the operation is said to be an allusion to 'the C-note or $100 bill, passed through world banks as money is laundered or rolled up and used to snort cocaine through the nose.' (Bush 1988: 9).

7 Referring to a slightly earlier period, Polich *et al*. (1984: 156–7) found that even a doubling of interdiction would have only limited effects on retail prices. See also Wagstaff and Maynard 1988.

8 The distinction between (i) level of organisation in the market (or an individual's importance in a local hierarchy) and (ii) the quantity of

drugs or persons seized is sometimes considered to be significant as one of the 'quality vs. quantity' indicators of the effectiveness of drugs policing. The most common quantity dimension is the number of arrests and officers do report pressure to produce such results. In this light, it is interesting that Trojanowicz (1990) – in advocating what he calls a 'community policing' approach – states that, 'Community Policing recognizes the folly of generating arrest statistics that look good on paper, but which fail to solve the problem. Community Officers do not shy away from making arrests, but they also understand that engaging the rest of the criminal justice system to little effect is not the answer' (1990: 23–4). This is part of a wider debate in the US about responses to drugs needing to focus on the causes, not just the symptoms (cf Eck (1989a) on the problem oriented approach); this argument has also been advanced by a Met Central Drugs Squad officer (Saltmarsh 1989). Another dimension to this 'causes not symptoms' approach goes under the name of 'demand reduction' which we look at in Chapter 7.

9 It should be noted that this is a rather idealised picture of the RCSs who in practice can be found to complain about many of the same issues that the area drugs squads do.

10 The informant played a role of 'vouching' – or giving a 'reference' – for the credibility of the undercover officer. This is akin to the procedure described as to 'duke in' an officer by an informant (Wilson 1978: 71). The informant then played no further part in this case.

11 Henry was an amphetamine supplier dealing in quantities of about one kilo a week. His supply route was established as delivering the kilo to a city in north east England, from where local dealers would do the rest. The police in that city confirmed that one kilo of amphetamine a week accounted for their entire problem with the drug. So by taking out the intermediary, the drugs squad had also 'stopped their complete amphetamine problem overnight'.

12 Cf Lyman's (1987: 99–101) advice on documenting cases and his 'record when you can' rule.

13 This 'taster' session is one of the critical moments for an officer working undercover, who would normally have to be seen to consume the drugs in order to maintain the identity (Williams and Guess 1981: 236). In this case it was to Trevor's advantage that because they met in a public place he had to go out of sight to pretend to sample the goods. There are obvious difficulties for officers posing as users. For example, Pritchard says he used a variety of techniques to give the appearance of consuming and rejected other drugs as not being ones he wanted to use (Pritchard and Laxton 1978: 85).

14 Both Garry and Colin (who appeared later to deliver the drugs) were known to the police as local villains but apparently neither were originally targets in this operation but came to notice through it. Garry did not stand trial at the time of this case (see Chapter 10) but was subsequently arrested in connection with this and another matter.

15 It should also be pointed out that demand reduction represents a move within the 'consumer countries' to demonstrate that the 'war on drugs' is not simply a one-sided affair in which the 'producer countries' are

being asked (or required) to take action against domestic production of coca leaves and opium.

16 The symbolism of the raids is complemented by the police penchant for spectacularly titled operations, suggesting an image of the police 'swooping'. For example, 'Operation Condor' in Brixton in 1987 and Operations 'Vulture' and 'Falcon' in Notting Hill in 1988.

17 In the event, out of the first twelve cases to be heard, one person was acquitted, with eleven being convicted. Four cases were pending at the time of writing.

18 William Bennett resigned as head of the Office of National Drug Control Policy in November 1990.

19 In Britain, drivers are being banned from driving for up to twelve months by the Driver and Vehicle Licensing Centre (DVLC) if a drug test proves positive (Bowcott 1990a: 1; *Police Review* 1990e: 1661). Cannabis is said to remain detectable for up to three months after it was taken, while other drugs like cocaine, amphetamines and opiates remain detectable for shorter periods.

20 CAT, launched in January 1988, is funded by a variety of sponsors and donations from private businesses, local government and the public. Its major sponsor, ADT – which in its 1988 Annual Report describes itself as the 'world's number one electronic security protection company', employing about 80,000 people across the world – has committed £1 million to it. ADT's chairman is also the chairman of the CAT Board of Trustees.

21 The Home Affairs Committee (1989b) had recommended that half the cost of payments to drug informants should be met from the centrally funded Common Police Services budget (*Police Review* 1989d: 2522). For the government response see Home Office 1990e: 13. In the US, TIP (Turn in a Pusher) programmes are described as moderately successful in getting information in exchange for money, including information from addicts anxious for money to purchase more drugs, who turn in dealers other than their own one (Williams and Guess 1981: 238; cf Marx 1988).

22 However, as the *Guardian*'s (editorial, 1990a: 18) more sober assessment pointed out, 'more money can be counter-productive'. There are at least three possible developments which would not be welcomed by the police: if the payments were successful in reducing the use of drugs, the price could be pushed up. But more worryingly, to guard against the possibility of having informants 'turning', criminal organisations may become likely to use – or at least to threaten to use – violence to seek to ensure confidentiality. 'The first big pay off is bound to be followed by violence to inhibit others from following the same path' (*ibid.*). A third possibility is that the potential promise of large rewards will increase the number of fraudulent leads being passed to the police. Although the system of classifying information according to the dependability of the informant will act as a screening system, the overall effect will be far more leads to follow up with no guarantee that any will prove to be more fruitful than under the current procedure.

23 Cf the account of the Garner/Lundy story by Jennings *et al.* (1990). 'On the eve of his [Garner's] trial he had met in secret with Lundy

and another senior officer to ask for help. The Met followed the usual procedure for secret informants and sent a letter to [the judge] Lowry asking for leniency. The judge was unimpressed' (*ibid.*: 111). Garner was jailed for four years, reduced on appeal to three years. In 1986 Garner was charged in connection with false passports: 'Again the Yard hierarchy secretly submitted a letter to the judge pleading for leniency. This time it worked and Garner's nine-month sentence ran concurrently with his fraud sentence. He did not have to serve one extra day in jail' (*ibid.*).

24 In the US the balance seems to have tipped over the other way. Raezer (1987: 41–2) reports on a Supreme Court ruling in 1980 that the *failure to cooperate* in identifying drug suppliers is a factor which can be considered when the court imposes a sentence. So the possibility of an increased sentence then becomes a further incentive to provide information.

25 Similarly Williams and Guess (1981: 238) refer to personal disputes as one of the best 'high yield' sources of information, but one which has to be acted on quickly in case the injured party has a change of heart.

26 The programme, based around the account of one of the Operation Albany investigators, was cancelled by the BBC following three written requests from Scotland Yard (Rose 1985a: 1; Leigh and Lashmar 1985: 1). The BBC later decided that the programme would never be transmitted (Rose 1985b: 6).

27 Marion Barry received a sentence of six months' imprisonment for the possession offence of which he was found guilty in October 1990.

28 The scope of the National Criminal Intelligence Service as anticipated by Ratcliffe included: all criminals of a national significance; all distinctive crime patterns; organised crime; animal rights; counterfeiters; drugs; peace convoys; public disorder; racial tensions; industrial arrest; itinerants; football hooliganism. Also, state security, for example 'the activities of anarchist groups which may influence operational policing. It is accepted that Special Branch [security police] will remain privy to detailed and sensitive information'. There would also be a 'reference section in respect of large scale operational matters, such as party political conferences, etc. The detailed planning for such events requires a very sound understanding of the techniques involved and the agencies capable of providing specialist advice.' And 'the role . . . at times of major outbreaks of public disorder or industrial action would be a natural extension of its functions which should encompass a permanent facility for monitoring such matters. A National Intelligence Office would become the intelligence wing of the Mutual Aid Coordinating Centre [an existing secretariat set up by Chief Constables which achieved prominence during the miners' strike of the early 1980s] at such times' (ACPO 1986: paras 6.12–6.14). Most, but not necessarily all, of these functions will eventually devolve to the National Criminal Intelligence Service when it becomes operational from 1992.

29 The Ratcliffe Report recommended the following indexes for the national database: nominal index (reference to all matters, subjects,

place names, person names, etc); vehicle index; crime index (abstract on every undetected serious crime), and 'crime series' (crimes linked by type of crime, geographical proximity, or officers' intuitive sense that there may be a link); and criminal methods (descriptions of particular techniques of committing offences) (ACPO 1986).

30 The committee to which the Coordinator of the National Criminal Intelligence Service will be responsible is expected to include representatives of the Home Office, the Foreign and Commonwealth Office, HM Customs and Excise, HM Inspectorate of Constabulary, the Association of Chief Police Officers, the Chair of ACPO's Crime Committee, ACPO Scotland, and the Assistant Commissioner of Special Operations (Metropolitan Police).

31 Powers of the Criminal Courts Act 1973, as amended by the DTOA section 32/6(1).

32 It may also be the case, but by no means is reliably established, that a convicted offender who continues to be 'cooperative' by naming other people as traffickers may be released from prison rather sooner than one who does not (or cannot). It seems not uncommon for enforcement personnel, who in reality have little to bargain with, to visit 'cooperative' convicted traffickers in the first few years of their confinement, to adopt a broadly sympathetic manner to prisoners' desire to be freed and, whilst not necessarily making clear suggestions that they would be able to facilitate an early release if further information is forthcoming, at least not to dash any expectations that this might be the case. An example of this sympathetic approach is given in the case of Roxanne, later in this chapter. In reality, in Britain, the scope for traffickers or any other convicted persons jailed for seven years or more to get bail before two thirds of their sentence has been served is severely restricted.

33 Even before the *Aramah* guidelines an 'appreciable' amount, with a retail value of less than £100,000, attracted a considerable sentence. For example, in the *Ashraf and Huq* case in 1982, Huq was found in possession of fifty-two grams of heroin said to be worth around £5,000, and received a sentence of ten years (Fortson 1988: 250).

34 For example, speaking at a conference organised by the Police Foundation in Cambridge in summer 1990, Commander John Grieve questioned the utility of war metaphors.

Bibliography

ACPO [Association of Chief Police Officers] (1975) *Report of the Sub-Committee on Criminal Intelligence* (Chairman, G.H. Baumber), unpublished.

ACPO (1985) *Final Report of the Working Party on Drugs Related Crime* (Chairman, R.F. Broome), unpublished; extracts in the Appendix to this book.

ACPO (1986) *Second Report of the Working Party on Operational Intelligence* (Chairman, A. Ratcliffe), unpublished.

Adler, P. (1985) *Wheeling and Dealing: An Ethnography of an Upper-level Drug Dealing and Smuggling Community*, New York: Columbia University Press.

Agar, M. (1978) 'When the Junk disappeared: Historical case of a heroin shortage', *Journal of Psychedelic Drugs* July–September, 10, 3: 255–61.

Alcoholism and Drug Abuse Week (1990) 'Court guidelines issued on denying benefits to drug users', 2, 37, 3 October: 7.

Anderson, M. (1989) *Policing the World*, Oxford: Clarendon.

Auld, J. (1981) *Marijuana Use and Social Control*, London: Academic Press.

Bakalar, J.B. and Grinspoon, L. (1984) *Drug Control in a Free Society*, Cambridge: Cambridge University Press.

Bamford, J. (1983) *The Puzzle Palace*, New York: Penguin.

Barnfield, C., Burns, S., Byrom, D.L. and Kemmenoe, A.V. (1988) 'The routine profiling for forensic heroin samples', *Forensic Science International* 39, 2: 107–17.

Bean, P. and Whynes, D.K. (1991) (eds) *Policing and Prescribing: The British System of Drug Control*, London: Macmillan, in press.

Bennett, W.J. (1989) 'Restoring authority', *New Perspectives Quarterly* 6, 2: 4–7.

Berridge, V. and Edwards, G. (1981) *Opium and the People: Opiate Use in Nineteenth-Century England*, London: Allen Lane.

Blok, A. (1974) *The Mafia of a Sicilian Village 1869–1960*, Oxford: Basil Blackwell.

Bottoms, A. (1983) 'Neglected features of contemporary penal systems', in D. Garland and P. Young (eds) *The Power to Punish: Contemporary Penality and Social Analysis*, Aldershot: Gower: 166–201.

Bowcott, O. (1989) 'Drug raid arrests spark clashes', *Guardian* 24 May: 24.

Bowcott, O. (1990a) 'Cannabis users face driving ban', *Guardian* 20 August: 1.

Bowcott, O. (1990b) 'Dangers may be rising with sentences', *Guardian* 20 August: 6.

Bruun, K., Pan, L. and Rexed, I. (1975) *The Gentlemen's Club: International Control of Drugs and Alcohol*, Chicago: University of Chicago Press.

Bucknall, P. and Ghodse, H. (1989) *Misuse of Drugs and Drug Trafficking Offences Act*, Supplement 3, London: Waterlow Publishers.

Buning, E., Drucker, E., O'Hare, P. and Newcombe, R. (eds) (1991) *Reduction of Drug Related Harm*, London: Routledge.

Burgess, R. (1984) *In the Field: An Introduction to Field Research*, London: Unwin Hyman.

Bush, J. (1988) 'The FBI spoilt the wedding', *Financial Times* 15 October: 9.

Campbell, D. (1990) *That was Business, this is Personal: The Changing Faces of Professional Crime*, London: Secker & Warburg.

Carvel, J. (1990) 'Foreign drug "mules" swell female jails' and 'Pawns in drug traffickers' game of chance', *Guardian* 30 July: 1 and 3.

Caseby, R. (1989) 'Riot estate drug gangs "tipped off"', *The Sunday Times* 1 October: 4.

Clutterbuck, R. (1990) *Terrorism, Drugs and Crime in Europe after 1992*, London: Routledge.

Cohen, S. (1979) 'The punitive city: notes on the dispersal of social control', *Contemporary Crises* 3: 339–63.

Commission of the European Communities (1990) DG Customs Union and Indirect Taxation, *Draft Proposal for a Council Regulation*, Brussels, 19 April.

Cook, S. (1990) 'No evidence against Yard commander, says DPP', *Guardian* 23 January: 3.

Cooper, B.M. (1987) 'Motor city breakdown', *Village Voice* 1 December: 23–35.

Cox, B., Shirley, J. and Short, M. (1977) *The Fall of Scotland Yard*, Harmondsworth: Penguin

Criminal Law Review (1983) 'Drug offences – sentencing guidelines; R. v. Aramah', April: 271–3.

Criminal Law Review (1987) 'R. v. Bilinski', November: 782–5.

Darbyshire, N. (1990), 'Is it time for an FBI in Britain?' *Daily Telegraph* 7 June: 19.

Davis, M. with Ruddick, S. (1988) 'Los Angeles: civil liberties between the hammer and the rock', *New Left Review* July–August, 170: 37–60.

Denniston, L. (1990a) 'Crackdown on buyers looks promising, study shows', *Drug Enforcement Report* 23 July: 5–6.

Denniston, L. (1990b) 'Government unlikely to abandon use of "stings"',

Drug Enforcement Report 23 August: 1–2.

Devalle, I. (1989) 'International movement of funds', *Drugs Arena* 7: 8–9

Didion, J. (1987) *Miami*, London: Weidenfeld & Nicolson.

Dodd-Crompton, A. (1990) 'Analytical techniques in investigating money laundering', *Drugs Arena* Autumn, 10: 2–8.

Dombrink, J. and Meeker, J. (1986) 'Beyond "Buy and Bust": nontraditional sanctions in federal drug law enforcement', *Contemporary Drug Problems* 13, 4: 711–40.

Dorn, N. (1983) *Alcohol, Youth and the State: Drinking Practices, Controls and Health Education*, London: Croom Helm.

Dorn, N. (1989) 'Reflections on two RAND reports', *International Journal on Drug Policy* November/December, 1, 3, 30–2

Dorn, N. (1991) 'Clarifying policy options on drug trafficking', in E. Buning, E. Drucker, P. O'Hare and R. Newcombe (eds) *Reduction of Drug Related Harm*, London: Routledge.

Dorn, N. and South, N. (1990) 'Drug Markets and Law Enforcement', *British Journal of Criminology* Spring, 30, 2: 171–188.

Dorn, N. and South, N. (1991) 'Profits and penalties: new trends in legislation and law enforcement concerning illegal drugs', in P. Bean and D. K. Whynes (eds) *Policing and Prescribing: The British System of Drug Control*, London: Macmillan.

Dorn, N., Murji, K. and South, N. (1991) 'Mirroring the market?', in R. Reiner and M. Cross (eds) *Beyond Law and Order*, London: Macmillan,

Downes, D. (1988) *Contrasts in Tolerance: Post-war Penal Policy in The Netherlands and England and Wales*, Oxford: Clarendon.

Drug Enforcement Administration (1982) *Narcotics Investigator's Manual*, Boulder, Colo: Paladin.

Drug Enforcement Administration and Royal Canadian Mounted Police (1988) *Money Laundering and the Illicit Drug Trade*, Washington, DC: DEA.

Drug Enforcement Report (1990a) 'New drug intelligence center set for possible startup in October', 25 June: 3.

Drug Enforcement Report (1990b) 'Bonner confirmation looks assured', 23 July: 6.

Drug Enforcement Report (1990c) 'Senate panel kills funding for intelligence center', 8 August: 1.

Druglink (1989) special issue on crack, 4, 5.

Drugs Arena (1990) 'Financial update', Spring, 9: 15.

Eck, J.E. (1989a) *Taking a Problem-Orientated Approach to Drug Enforcement*, Washington, DC: Police Executive Research Forum.

Eck, J.E. (1989b) 'The future of drug control efforts', paper prepared for Future Issues in Policing: A Working Symposium, Canadian Police College, Ottawa, Ontario, 27–29 June.

The Economist (1989) 'Laundering money – whitewash or crackdown', reprinted in *Drugs Arena* 7.

Fagan, J. (1989) 'The social organisation of drug use and drug dealing among urban gangs', *Criminology* November, 27, 4: 633–67.

Feldman, H., Mandel, J. and Fields, A. (1985) 'In the neighbourhood: a strategy for delivering early intervention services to young drug users in their natural environments', in A. Friedman and G. Beschner (eds) *Treatment Services for Adolescent Substance Users*, Rockville, Md: NIDA.

File on Four (1990) 'Crack on the front line', BBC Radio 4 documentary, 10 April, transcript.

Fortson, R. (1988) *The Law on the Misuse of Drugs*, London: Sweet & Maxwell.

Foster, J. (1990) *Villains*, London: Routledge.

Foucault, M. (1977) *Discipline and Punish: The Birth of the Prison*, London: Allen Lane.

Fraser, A. and George, M. (1988) 'Changing trends in drug use: an initial follow-up of a local heroin using community', *British Journal of Addiction* 83, 6: 655–63.

Fryer, P. (1984) *Staying Power: The History of Black People in Britain*, London: Pluto.

Fuqua, P. (1978) *Drug Abuse: Investigation and Control*, New York: McGraw-Hill.

García Márquez, G. (1990) 'The future of Colombia', *Granta 31*, London: Penguin: 86–95.

George, M. and Fraser, A. (1989) 'Changing trends in drug use: a second follow-up of a local heroin using community', *British Journal of Addiction* 84, 12: 1,461–6.

Gillard, M. (1988) 'BCCI: the cocaine cash trail', *Observer* 16 October: 56.

Gilman, M. and Pearson, G. (1991) 'Lifestyles and law enforcement', in P. Bean and D.K. Whynes (eds) *Policing and Prescribing: The British System of Drug Control*, London: Macmillan.

Glaser, B. and Strauss, A. (1967) *The Discovery of Grounded Theory: Strategies for Qualitative Research*, Chicago: Aldine.

Graef, R. (1990) 'All saints and sinners', *ES* (*Evening Standard* magazine) 22 August: 22–8.

Grannatt, M. (1989) 'Broadwater Farm and the media', *Police Review* 20 October: 2, 124–5.

Grieve, J. (1987) 'Comparative police strategies – drug related crime', unpublished MPhil thesis, Cranfield Institute of Technology.

Guardian (1990a) 'Super for grasses', editorial, 15 February: 18.

Guardian (1990b) 'A touch too acid', editorial, 4 July: 18.

Hall, S., Critcher, C., Jefferson, T., Clarke, J. and Roberts, B. (1978) *Policing the Crisis: mugging, the state and law and order*, London: Macmillan.

Harvey, L. and Pease, K. (1987) 'Guideline judgments and proportionality in sentencing', *Criminal Law Review* February: 96–104.

Hecker, S. and Kaplan, M. (1989) 'Workplace drug testing as social control', *International Journal of Health Services* 19, 4: 693–707.

Henry, S. (1978) *The Hidden Economy*, Oxford: Martin Robertson.

Herbert, S. (1989) 'An expedient of last resort', *Guardian* law report, 22 July: 21.

The Hill (1989) 'The Bill on the Hill', 51, February: 7–8.

Hilliard, B. (1989) '"Blacked" by computer', *Police Review* 15 December: 2537.

Hobbs, D. (1988) *Doing the Business: Entrepreneurship, the Working Class and Detectives in the East End of London*, Oxford: Clarendon.

Hodgson, D., Nicol, A., Blom-Cooper, L., Iredale, M., Leifer, N.A., Sewell, J.M., Soley, C., Staughton, C. and Walker, N. (1984) *The Profits of Crime and their Recovery*, London: Heinemann.

Holdaway, S. (1989) 'Discovering structure. Studies of the British police occupational culture', in M. Weatheritt (ed.) *Police Research: Some Future Prospects*, Aldershot: Avebury.

Home Affairs Committee (1985) *Misuse of Hard Drugs*, interim report, London: HMSO.

Home Affairs Committee (1989a) *Crack: The Threat of Hard Drugs in the Next Decade*, interim report, London: HMSO.

Home Affairs Committee (1989b) *Drug Trafficking and Related Serious Crime*, London: HMSO.

Home Affairs Committee (1990) *Practical Police Cooperation in the European Community*, London: HMSO.

Home Office (1990a) *Crime, Justice and Protecting the Public: The Government's Proposals for Legislation*, London: HMSO.

Home Office (1990b) *UK Action on Drug Misuse: The Government's Strategy*, London: HMSO.

Home Office (1990c) 'Organisers of illegal acid house parties face tough new penalties', news release, 13 July.

Home Office (1990d) 'Illegal acid house party organisers face confiscation of profits', news release, 24 August.

Home Office (1990e) *The Government Response to the Seventh Report of the Home Affairs Committee Session 1988–89 (HC 370) Drug Trafficking and Related Serious Crime, and the Sixth (Interim) report (HC 356) Crack: The Threat of Hard Drugs in the Next Decade*, London: HMSO.

Horsnell, M. (1988) 'Drug gang jailed for smuggling cannabis worth £4m into UK', *The Times* 16 September: 3.

Hoyland, P. (1989) 'Police accused over drugs raid riot', *Guardian* 25 May: 2.

Hughes, P.H., Crawford, G.A., Barker, N.W., Schumann, S. and Jaffe, J.H. (1971) 'The social structure of a heroin copping community', *American Journal of Psychiatry* November, 128: 551–8.

ICPO General Secretariat (1989) 'The diversion of chemicals and the clandestine manufacture of drugs', *International Criminal Police Review* 417, March–April: 18–27.

ICPR [*International Criminal Police Review*] (1989b) 'Hawala banking – A money laundering system', 418, May–June: 28.

Imbert, P. (1989) 'Crimes without frontiers', *Police Review*, 9 June: 1,174–5.

IRR: Police–Media Research Project (1990) 'Notting Hill inquiry findings to be "suppressed"', Bulletin 62, 18 June–22 July: 2–3.

Jennings, A., Lashmar, P. and Simson, V. (1990) *Scotland Yard's Cocaine Connection*, London: Jonathan Cape.

Johnson, B. (1980) 'Toward a theory of drug subcultures', in D.J. Lettieri, M. Sayers and H.W. Pearson (eds) *Theories on Drug Abuse*, NIDA Research Monograph 30, Rockville, Md: NIDA.

Johnson, B. (1989) 'Crime and compulsory treatment', *Druglink* May–June 4, 3: 12–13.

Johnson, B., Goldstein, P., Preble, E., Schmeidler, J., Lipton, D.S., Spunt, B. and Miller, T. (1985) *Taking Care of Business: The Economics of Crime by Heroin Abusers*, Lexington, Mass: D.C. Heath.

Kay, L. (1988) 'Aramah and the street value of drugs', *Criminal Law Review* December: 814–20.

Keith, M. (1986) 'The 1981 Riots in London', DPhil thesis, University of Oxford.

Kirby, T. (1989a) 'Wife cleared of helping drugs smuggler to escape', *Independent* 22 April: 5.

Kirby, T. (1989b) 'Police accused of planting drugs on blacks', *Independent* 17 June: 5.

Kirby, T. (1989c) 'The party's over in an Acid House under the arches', *Independent* 22 August: 5.

Kleiman, M.A.R. (1989) *Marijuana: Costs of Abuse, Costs of Control*, New York: Greenwood Press

Langer, J. (1977) 'Drug entrepreneurs and dealing culture', *Social Problems* 24, 3: 377–86.

Lawn, J.C. (1985) 'The DEA's role in the prevention of drug trafficking and abuse', *The Police Chief* October, LII, 10: 31–41.

Leigh, D. (1989) 'Revealed: Yard held up drug hunt', *Observer* 2 May: 3.

Leigh, D. and Lashmar, P. (1985) 'BBC exposé halted by Yard pressure', *Observer* 13 October: 1.

Levin, B. (1990a) 'Justice under a blue cloud', *The Times* 12 January: 14.

Levin, B. (1990b) 'What more evidence must they have?', *The Times* 25 January: 12.

Lewis, R. (1989) 'European markets in cocaine', *Contemporary Crises* 13: 35–52.

Lewis, R., Hartnoll, R., Bryer, S., Daviaud, E. and Mitcheson, M. (1985) 'Scoring smack: The illicit heroin market in London 1980–1983', *British Journal of Addiction* 80, 3: 281–90.

Lichfield, J. (1989) 'Bush targets users in new drug fight', *Independent* 17 August: 6.

Lundy, T. (1989) 'The truth behind the report', *Police Review* 4 August: 1,574.

Lyman, M.D. (1987) *Narcotics and Crime Control*, Springfield, Ill.: C.C. Thomas.

McCoy, A. (1974) 'The politics of the poppy in Indochina', in L. Simmonds and A. Said (eds) *Drugs, Politics and Diplomacy: The International Connection*, Beverly Hills, Calif: Sage.

McCoy, A. Read, C. and Adams, L. (1972) *The Politics of Heroin in Southeast Asia*, New York: Harper & Row.

McDermott, Q. (1989) 'Siege mentality', *City Limits* no. 409, 3–10 August: 7.

McNichol, T. (1990) 'The high times and low life of Mayor Marion Barry',

Guardian weekend section 3–4 February: 12–13.

Manning, P.K. (1980) *The Narcs' Game: Organizational and Informational Limits on Drug Law Enforcement*, Cambridge, Mass: MIT Press.

Manning, P.K. and Redlinger, L.J. (1978) 'Working bases for corruption: Organizational ambiguities and narcotics law enforcement', in A.S. Trebach (ed.) *Drugs, Crime and Politics*, New York: Praeger, pp 60–89.

Marriott, M. (1989) 'New York's worst drug sites: markets of death and despair', *New York Times* 1 June: 1–4.

Marx, G.T. (1988) *Undercover: Police Surveillance in America*, Berkeley: University of California Press.

Mathiesen, T. (1980) 'The future of control systems – the case of Norway', *International Journal of the Sociology of Law* 8: 149–64.

Mieczkowski, T. (1986) 'Geeking up and throwing down: heroin street life in Detroit', *Criminology* 24: 645–66.

Moore. M.H. (1977) *Buy and Bust: The Effective Regulation of an Illicit Market in Heroin*, Lexington, Mass: Lexington Books.

Moore, M.H. and Kleiman, M.A.R. (1989) *The Police and Drugs*, Washington, DC: National Institute of Justice.

Morton, J. (1989) 'Will the parties soon be over?', *Police Review* 20 October: 2,120–1.

NDIU [National Drugs Intelligence Unit] (1989), memorandum submitted to the Home Affairs Committee (1989b) *Drug Trafficking and Related Serious Crime*, vol. 2, London: HMSO.

NDIU (nd) *The United Kingdom National Drugs Intelligence Unit*, London: NDIU.

Office of National Drug Control Policy (1989) *National Drug Control Strategy*, Washington, DC: Executive Office of the President.

Parker, H., Bakx, K. and Newcombe, R. (1988) *Living with Heroin: The Impact of a Drugs 'Epidemic' on an English Community*, Milton Keynes: Open University Press.

Pearson, G. (1987) *The New Heroin Users*, Oxford: Basil Blackwell.

Pearson, G. (1989) 'The street connection', *New Statesman & Society* 15 September: 10–11.

Pearson, G. (1991) 'Drugs and criminal justice: a harm reduction* perspective', in E. Buning, E. Drucker, P. O'Hare and R. Newcombe (eds) *Reduction of Drug Related Harm*, London: Routledge.

Pistone, J.D. and Woodley, R. (1988) *Donnie Brasco: my undercover life in the mafia*, London: Pan.

Police Review (1989a) 'Crack raid sparks riot in Wolverhampton', 26 May: 1,055.

Police Review (1989b) 'MP urges confiscation of acid house party profits', 27 October: 2,166.

Police Review (1989c) 'Acid party organiser convicted', 17 November: 2,314.

Police Review (1989d) 'Central funds for drug informants', 15 December: 2,522.

Police Review (1990a) 'Three-year inquiry clears Commander', 26 January: 166.

Police Review (1990b) 'Bank secrecy waived after laundering scandal', 16 February: 325.

Police Review (1990c) 'Money laundering to be made a crime throughout Europe', 2 March: 429.

Police Review (1990d) 'National police chief for new intelligence unit', 27 July: 1,478.

Police Review (1990e) 'Drugged-driving bans increase', 24 August: 1661.

PERF [Police Executive Research Forum] (1986) 'Proposal for research on strategies for incapacitating narcotics wholesalers', submitted to National Institute of Justice, Washington, DC: PERF

Polich, J.M., Ellickson, P.L., Reuter, P. and Kahan, J.P. (1984) *Strategies for Controlling Adolescent Drug Use*, Santa Monica, Calif: RAND.

Preble, E and Casey, J, 1969, 'Taking care of business: the heroin users' life on the street', *International Journal of the Addictions* 4, 1: 1–24.

Price, B. (1989) Verbal evidence in Volume 2 of Home Affairs Committee (1989b) *Drug Trafficking and Related Serious Crime*, London: HMSO.

Pringle, P. (1990) 'Barry seeks to "heal my body, mind and soul"', *Independent* 22 January: 10.

Pritchard, M. and Laxton, E. (1978) *Busted! The Sensational Life Story of an Undercover Hippie Cop*, London: Mirror Books.

Punch, M. (1985) *Conduct Unbecoming: The Social Construction of Police Deviance*, London: Tavistock.

Raezer, T.A. (1987) 'Needed weapons in the Army's war on drugs: electronic surveillance and informants', *Military Law Review* 116: 1–65.

Reiner, R. (1985) *The Politics of the Police*, Brighton: Wheatsheaf.

Reuter, P. (1983) *Disorganised Crime: Illegal Markets and the Mafia*, Cambridge, Mass: MIT Press.

Reuter, P. and Haaga, J. (1989) *The Organization of High-Level Drug Markets: An Exploratory Study*, Santa Monica, Calif: RAND.

Reuter, P., Crawford, G. and Cave, J. (1988) *Sealing the Borders: The Effects of Increased Military Participation in Drug Interdiction*, Santa Monica, Calif: RAND.

Reuter, P., MacCoun, R. and Murphy, P. (1990) *Money from Crime: A Study of the Economics of Drug Dealing in Washington, D.C.*, Santa Monica, Calif: RAND.

Rose, D. (1985a) 'BBC film stopped after three police requests', *Guardian* 14 October: 1.

Rose, D. (1985b) 'Documentary on organised crime ditched by BBC', *Guardian*, 15 October: 6.

Rose, D. (1988) 'Great Train Robbers dealt cocaine', *Guardian* 27 July: 8.

Ruggiero, V. (1990a) 'I mercati della droga in Italia e Gran Bretagna', *Inchiesta* gennaio–marzo, 87: 59–67.

Ruggiero, V. (1990b) 'L'Eroina a Londra e a Torino: Uno Studio Comparativo', PhD thesis, Universita di Bologna.

Rusche, G. and Kirchheimer, O. (1939) *Punishment and Social Structure*, New York: Russell & Russell.

Sagarin, E. and McNamara, D. (1972) 'The problem of entrapment', in R. Dahl and G. Dix (eds) *Crime Law and Justice Annual 1972*, Buffalo,

NY: W.S. Hein.

Saltmarsh, G. (1989) *Alternatives in the disposition and management of assets seized from drug traffickers and other major criminals: a report of the findings of a study in the United States and Britain*, London: Winston Churchill Memorial Trust.

Sapsted, D. (1989) 'Police intelligence unit to fight acid house lawlessness, *The Times* 17 October: 2.

Seton, C. (1990) 'Drugs case dropped to protect informant', *The Times* 13 June: 3.

Sharrock, D. (1990) 'New police squad to fight serious crime', *Guardian* 7 June: 3.

Skolnick, J.H. (1966) *Justice Without Trial: Law Enforcement in Democratic Society*, New York: Wiley.

Skolnick, J.H. (1984) 'The limits of narcotics law enforcement', *Journal of Psychoactive Drugs* April–June, 16, 2: 119–27.

South, N. (1988) *Policing for Profit*, London: Sage.

Stern, C. (1989) 'How leaks grew on the farm', *Police Review* 13 October: 2,070–1.

Stewart, T. (1987) *The Heroin Users*, London: Pandora.

Sweeney, J. (1989) 'Heirs to the Krays', *Observer Magazine* 25 June: 27–30.

Sweeney, J. (1990) 'Silencing of the silent man', *Observer* 29 April: 19.

Tan, Y.H. (1989) 'Public interest in disclosing informer's identity', *Independent* 4 August: 16.

Taylor, L. (1984) *In the Underworld*, Oxford: Basil Blackwell.

Tendler, S. (1988) 'Drug gangsters jailed over big amphetamine "factory"', *The Times* 21 September: 3.

Tendler, S. (1989) 'Supergrass gets 22 years for smuggling in cocaine', *The Times* 24 March: 5.

Thompson, M. (1989) 'Los Angeles police barricade neighborhood to stop drug dealing', *Drug Enforcement Report* 8 December: 8.

Tisdall, S. (1990) 'Sting in the tail of Barry saga', *Guardian* 27 January: 6.

Trojanowicz, R. (1990) 'Community policing and drugs: new directions in the U.S. national drug strategy', paper presented to a conference on Drug Misuse in Local Communities: Perspectives across Europe, Cambridge, 7–10 September.

US Comptroller General (1976) *Difficulties in Immobilizing Major Narcotics Traffickers*, reprinted in US Congress, Senate Committee on the Judiciary, Subcommittee to investigate juvenile delinquency, *The Narcotic Sentencing and Seizure Act of 1976: Hearings before the Subcommittee*, Washington, DC: GPO.

US General Accounting Office (1984) *Investigations of Major Drug Trafficking Organizations*, Washington, DC: GAO.

US SFRC [Senate Foreign Relations Committee] Subcommittee on Narcotics and Terrorism (1990) 'Drug money laundering, banks and foreign policy', a report to the Foreign Relations Committee on 27 September and 4 October, Washington, DC: US Government Printing Office.

Wagstaff, A. and Maynard, A. (1988) *Economic Aspects of the Illicit Drug*

Market and Drug Enforcement Policies in the United Kingdom, Home Office Research Study 95, London: HMSO.

Wainwright, M. (1990) '800 arrested in acid house raid', *Guardian* 23 July: 1.

Ward, S. (1989) 'Police "used undue force" to control street fighting', *Independent* 25 May: 3.

Warner, J. (1990) 'Undercover investigations: the need for policy,* coordination and control', *Narcotics Control Digest* 20, 20: 1–5.

Waymont, A. and Wright, A. (1989) *Drug Enforcement Strategies and Intelligence Needs*, unpublished draft, London: Police Foundation.

Williams, J.R. and Guess, L.L. (1981) 'The informant: a narcotics enforcement dilemma', *Journal of Psychoactive Drugs* July–September, 13, 3: 235–45.

Williams, J.R., Redlinger L.J. and Manning, P.K. (1979) *Police Narcotics Control: Patterns and Strategies*, summary, Washington, DC: US Department of Justice.

Williams, T. (1989) *The Cocaine Kids: The Inside Story of a Teenage Drug Ring*, Reading, Mass: Addison-Wesley.

Willis, P. (1978) *Profane Culture*, London: Routledge & Kegan Paul.

Wilson, J.Q. (1978) *The Investigators: Managing FBI and Narcotics Agents*, New York: Basic Books.

Wilson, J.Q. (1985) *Thinking About Crime*, revised edition, New York: Vintage Books.

Wisotsky, S. (1987) 'Crackdown: the emerging "drug exception" to the Bill of Rights', *Hastings Law Journal* July, 38, 5: 889–926.

Woodiwiss, M. (1988) *Crime Crusades and Corruption: Prohibition in the United States 1900–1987*, London: Pinter.

Zander, M. (1989) *Confiscation and Forfeiture Law: English and American Comparisons*, London: Police Foundation.

Zimmer, L. (1987) *Operation Pressure Point: The Disruption of Street-Level Drug Trade on New York's Lower East Side*, New York: Center for Research in Crime and Justice, NY University School of Law.

Name index

Subject index